Real RDAs
for
Real People

Real RDAs
for
Real People

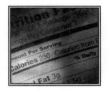

Why "Official" Nutrition Guidelines
Aren't Enough and
What To Do About It

Mike Fillon

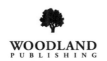

WOODLAND
PUBLISHING

The CIP record for this book is available from the Library of Congress.

For ordering information, contact:
Woodland Publishing, 448 East 800 North, Orem, Utah 84097
(800) 777-2665

The information in this book is for educational purposes only and is not recommended as a means of diagnosing or treating an illness. All matters concerning physical and mental health should be supervised by a health practitioner knowledgeable in treating that particular condition. Neither the publisher nor author directly or indirectly dispenses medical advice, nor do they prescribe any remedies or assume any responsibility for those who choose to treat themselves.

ISBN 1-58054-356-1

Printed in the United States of America
Please visit our Web site:
www.woodlandpublishing.com

for Sue

Contents

Foreword

Every once in a while a book comes along with a message that's a true wake-up call, a book that not only cuts through the politics of a given topic, but also clearly explains those politics as well.

Such is the case with many of today's nutritional problems. Willing to spill the beans concerning the influence of some very powerful food interests, Mike Fillon tells it the way it is concerning some very important issues dogging us today—the inadequacies of our "official" nutrition guidelines (including the food pyramid), the influence of money and politics on science, the prevalence of sugar in our diet, and many other important topics.

Real RDAs for Real People is not a "single issue" book—thank heavens. It's a broad exposé of dangers we all need to be aware of as we try to determine the best course of action trying to stay healthy. Furthermore, we learn within these pages that some information sources that appear both reliable and unbiased are not always so.

As a matter of fact, that may be the most valuable lesson this book teaches us. There's big money out there with a vested interest in getting us to consume foods that may be great for its company's bottom line, but not so great for our bottoms (or our tickers, or a variety of other organs). Having the insight to see through an organization's motives is worth more than all the herbal tea in China— and certainly worth the price of this book. It's vital to realize that prevalent medical and nutritional science and research are influenced (and even coerced) by research-funding organizations and lobby groups pushing their own agendas and affiliations.

More and more of us are becoming aware that something is wrong with the way our food industries and our health care system operate. We're far fatter than ever before, even while trying so hard to consume less fat. Heart disease is on the increase. Cancer is on the increase. Diabetes cases are skyrocketing. And we're told we live in the most advanced health care system in the world? You're about to discover that our government's nutrition guidelines, as they now stand, are unsatisfactory for several reasons. In addition to learning what those reasons are, *Real RDAs* provides current, detailed information on the human body's real needs for and tolerances of every major nutrient. This list is much bigger than the required list on food labels, including everything from macronutrients like protein, carbohydrates, fat, and fiber to micronutrients like vitamins, minerals, phytochemicals and flavonoids.

We should be learning the points in this book from other sources, but we aren't. Finding out exactly why we aren't seems to be a pretty difficult task, but there's something fishy going on in Washington. We're not getting straight answers from the U.S. Department of Agriculture or the FDA, and we especially don't get straight answers from food lobbies and private interest groups who fund most of today's research. We don't get the full story from CNN or the morning paper. Maybe they're incapable of revealing that information; maybe they have reason not to reveal it.

Either way, you came to the right place. Many of those answers are within these pages. In a world of ever-more-confusing alphabet soup of RDAs, RDIs, DRIs, DVs, IFICs, CCFs, ACSHs and many others (whew!), Mike Fillon cuts through the muck, telling us both what the message is, and who's giving it to us. Included are easy-to-read tables and new, more accurate, more helpful nutrition guidelines based on age, gender and ethnic background. These are "need-to-know" messages if you want to stay healthy.

If I didn't know better, I'd think I wrote some of these chapters myself. That doesn't necessarily make them good, of course, but it does mean that some of the messages I've tried to get across to patients, athletes, and readers for over twenty years are being reinforced here . . . and that makes my day.

Read, learn, and enjoy.

Allan N. Spreen, M.D.

Part I

Alphabet Goop

Our nutritional guidelines have evolved into a confusing string of initials representing meaningless, confusing descriptions. Developed with the greatest intentions—and we all know where that paved road leads—any help they offer is buried in scientific jargon; rendering the help and guidance they promise too confusing and certainly not followed.

There's an old saying that too many cooks spoil the broth. This certainly applies to our nation's nutritional guidelines, which have been unduly influenced by lobby groups and food companies who have pushed to season our collective broth with too many sweets along with salt and fat. The result? Many of us are gobbling up way too many calories, growing obese as the rates of diabetes, hypertension and heart disease skyrocket.

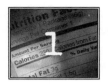

We're All Just Average

Although we've probably never met, there's one thing I do know about you; when it comes to nutritional advice and your health, the U.S. government thinks you're average—very, very average. It doesn't matter how tall you are, what your gender is, or, until recently, even how much you weigh. Your age or the environment where you live doesn't matter all that much either—you're average.

Before you get all huffy, you should know they think the same thing about your next-door neighbors and your aunt Tallulah in Topeka. You say you don't have an aunt Tallulah in Topeka? Doesn't matter. Regardless of what your aunt's name is and where she lives, her nutritional needs are considered average. Frankly, they think the same about me, and that doesn't thrill me either.

In 1894, the U.S. Department of Agriculture (USDA) published its first dietary recommendations based on a *Farmers' Bulletin* written by W. O. Atwater, the USDA's director of the Office of Experiment Stations. At the time, specific vitamins and minerals hadn't even been discovered, and most illnesses were blamed on germs, not nutritional deficiencies. Atwater was the first to believe that food composition, diet and health were connected, and he set out to prove it scientifically.

In 1916, the UDSA published the first food guide, *Food for Young Children*, by Caroline Hunt. She categorized foods into five groups:

- milk and meats
- cereals
- vegetables and fruits
- fats and fatty foods
- sugars and sugary foods

The next year, Hunt teamed up with Atwater to publish *How to Select Foods*, based on these five groups. In 1921, a guide recommending what food to purchase for the average family of five was published. Throughout the rest of the 1920s and 1930s, new food buying guides—based on different family sizes and incomes—were developed and based upon twelve major food groups. Again, income and family sizes were the overriding factors in the development of these food groups.

In 1941, at the urging of President Franklin Roosevelt, the first Recommended Daily Allowances (RDA) for vitamins and minerals were devised—as a means of ensuring that American Soldiers in World War II received rations that would prevent severe nutritional deficiencies such as beriberi and scurvy. The government defined RDAs as the levels of intake of essential nutrients judged to be adequate to meet the known needs of practically all healthy persons.

At the time, it was generally believed all people needed similar amounts of calories and nine essential nutrients. The nutrients on the list were:

- protein
- iron
- calcium
- vitamin A
- vitamin D
- thiamin (vitamin B1)
- riboflavin (vitamin B2)
- niacin (vitamin B3)
- ascorbic acid (vitamin C)

Since 1941, the Food and Nutrition Board (FNB) of the National Academy of Sciences (NAS) and the USDA have updated the RDAs ten times. The most recent revision was in 1989 when RDAs were determined for protein, eleven vitamins, and seven minerals.

In 1995, the FNB decided a new, more comprehensive approach was necessary in setting dietary guidelines. Research showed that higher intakes of some nutrients promote health and prevents chronic disease. The FNB also recognized rapid growth in food fortification by the food industry and in the use of dietary supplements. They also realized the existing RDAs did not adequately distinguish guidelines for "population groups" from those for individuals.

So, the Board replaced and expanded the current RDAs with what they decided to call Dietary Reference Intakes or DRIs. The DRIs are actually a set of four reference values:

Recommended Dietary Allowance (RDA) is the average daily dietary intake of a nutrient that is sufficient to meet the requirement of nearly all (97–98 percent) healthy persons. They used to stand alone, but are now one factor in the broader, more confusing DRIs.

Adequate Intake (AI) for a nutrient is established only when an RDA cannot be determined. Therefore, a nutrient either has an RDA or an AI. The AI is based on observed intakes of the nutrient by a group of healthy persons.

Tolerable Upper Intake Level (UL) is the highest daily intake of a nutrient that is likely to pose no risks of toxicity for almost all individuals. As intake above the UL increases, risk increases.

Estimated Average Requirement (EAR) is the amount of a nutrient that is estimated to meet the requirement for half of all healthy individuals in the population.

For the most part, each of these reference values distinguishes between gender and broadly defined life stages. While RDAs, AIs and ULs are intended as dietary guidelines for individuals, EARs provide guidelines for groups and populations. In addition, factors that might modify these guidelines, such as availability of nutrients from different sources, nutrient-nutrient and nutrient-drug interactions, and the impact from food fortified by nutrients and supplements, are incorporated into the guidelines in much greater detail than previous standards.

While the DRIs are a big improvement over the RDAs—at least on paper—they still fall vastly short in telling us very much, as you'll see in the next chapter.

Establishing the DRIs has been a huge undertaking requiring more than five years of research so far and involving several panels of independent experts to evaluate the data. And they're not done yet. Once all the initial DRIs are established, the U.S. government intends to update them regularly as new data becomes available and as scientists continue to study individual nutrients.

In addition to providing information for labels on food (known as RDIs), RDAs—and now the DRIs—are used for many other purposes. For example, schools, prisons, hospitals and nursing homes use the RDAs to plan healthful diets. Also, the food industry uses RDAs to develop new food products. Policy makers use them to evaluate and improve food supplies to meet national needs. Health workers also use them to provide nutrition education.

So then, what's the problem? There are many, as you'll see in the next chapter. Before I go on, it might be helpful if I provided a few definitions.

Vitamins

Vitamins are complex organic substances that are needed in very small amounts for many of the processes carried out in the body. Usually only a few milligrams (mg) or micrograms (mcg) are needed per day, but these amounts are essential for health. Most vitamins cannot be made by the body, so they have to be provided by the diet. Two exceptions are D, which can be obtained by the action of sunlight on the skin, and small amounts of a B vitamin niacin, which can be made from the amino acid tryptophan.

Vitamins have a variety of functions in the body: some are cofactors in enzyme activity, some are antioxidants (preventing oxygen from doing damage in the body) and one (vitamin D) is a prohormone. If insufficient amounts of vitamins are available to the body because of a poor diet or some medical condition (e.g., malabsorption), certain symptoms will appear and can develop into a deficiency disease. Vitamin deficiency diseases are rare in the U.S. but still occur in some parts of the world.

Vitamins have been traditionally grouped into two categories: the fat-soluble vitamins, and the water-soluble vitamins.

Minerals

Minerals are naturally occurring elements found in the earth's soil. When we eat fresh fruits and vegetables, we get trace minerals from the soil in which the fruits and vegetables were grown; when we eat beef or chicken, we get trace minerals from the hay or feed of the animal.

Minerals act as coenzymes enabling the body to perform its functions, including energy production, growth, and healing. Basically, there are two types of minerals: bulk and trace. Bulk minerals such as calcium, magnesium, sodium, and potassium are needed in larger amounts than trace minerals such as boron, chromium, copper, iodine, iron, manganese, selenium, and zinc. Since minerals are stored in the body's bone and muscle tissue, it is possible to develop toxicity, but only if megadoses are taken over a prolonged period of time.

Micronutrients

Micronutrients are substances needed by the body in very small amounts. Most are not made by the human body and must be provided by food. These micronutrients are essential for the body to maintain its normal functions. Without them, the body cannot function optimally and different health problems occur. If micronutrients are missing during phases of rapid growth, the development of basic biological functions like intellect, and even life itself, can be threatened. This is why young children and pregnant women are often among the risk groups for micronutrient deficiencies.

All vitamins and most minerals are micronutrients. Deficiencies in some of these micronutrients eventually give rise to specific and recognizable signs, for example, lack of iodine can cause an enlarged thyroid gland (goiter), recognizable by the unsightly swelling on the throat. Other deficiencies may cause more general signs such as weakness, paleness and lack of resistance to infections.

The three major micronutrient deficiencies emphasized by the World Health Organization (WHO) worldwide are vitamin A, iron and iodine deficiencies.

Macronutrients

All foods are composed of three macronutrients: carbohydrates, protein and fat. Some foods are primarily carbohydrate (bread); others are mainly protein (turkey), and some are pure fat (olive oil). Other foods are combinations of two or all three. In order to properly function, your body needs all three of these macronutrients in approximately the following ratio: 55 percent carbohydrates, 15 percent protein and no more than 30 percent total fat.

Since I'll be mentioning the following items frequently in the next several chapter, I think it's worth it to go over them one more time.

DRI

The DRIs, or Dietary Reference Intakes, is an umbrella group that includes the old stand-alone RDAs and the AIs (Adequate Intakes), EARs (Estimated Average Requirements) and ULs (Tolerable Upper Intakes). Many of the nutrients have been switched to DRIs. These will eventually take the place of the RDAs.

RDA

The RDAs were developed for healthy people under "normal" circumstances (i.e., no illness, no genetic weaknesses, no exposure to environmental toxins) to prevent the development of overt deficiency diseases. RDAs were not developed to serve as a guide to determining optimal nutritional needs.

RDI

On January 1, 1997, The U.S. Food and Drug Administration (FDA) began phasing in new labeling requirements—which are now official. One of the changes that has caused some confusion is the switch from Recommended Daily Allowance (RDA) to Recommended Daily Intake (RDI). Also, vitamin and mineral listings on food labels are now followed by Percentage of Daily Value (%DV).

Table 1.1 Vitamins: Comparisons Over Time, 1968 to Present

VITAMIN	RDI*	1968 RDA†	1974 RDA†	1980 RDA†	1989 RDA†	DRIs‡
Vitamin A	5,000 IU	5,000 IU	5,000 IU	5,000 IU	5,000 IU	3,000 IU
Vitamin C	60 mg	60 mg	45 mg	60 mg	60 mg	90 mcg
Vitamin D	10 mcg	10 mcg	10 mcg	10 mcg	10 mcg	15 mcg
Vitamin E	20 mg	20 mg	10 mg	10 mg	10 mg	15 mg§
Vitamin K	80 mcg	--	--	70–140 mcg	80 mcg	120 mcg
Thiamin	1.5 mg	1.5 mg	1.5 mg	1.5 mg	1.5 mg	1.2 mg
Riboflavin	1.7 mg	1.7 mg	1.8 mg	1.7 mg	1.8 mg	1.3 mg
Niacin	20 mg	20 mg	20 mg	19 mg	20 mg	16 mg
Vitamin B-6	2 mg	2 mg	2 mg	2.2 mg	2 mg	1.7 mg
Folate	400 mcg	400 mcg	400 mcg	400 mcg	200 mcg	400 mcg#
Vitamin B-12	6 mcg	6 mcg	3 mcg	3 mcg	2 mcg	2.4 mcg**
Biotin	300 mcg	150–300 mcg	100–300 mcg	100–200 mcg	30–100 mcg	30 mcg
Pantothenic	10 mg	5–10 mg	5–10 mg	4-7 mg	4-7 mg	5 mg
Choline	--	--	--	--	--	550 mg

* The Reference Daily Intake (RDI) is the value established by the Food and Drug Administration (FDA) for use in nutrition labeling. It was based initially on the highest 1968 Recommended Dietary Allowance (RDA) for each nutrient, to assure that needs were met for all age groups.

† The RDAs were established and periodically revised by the Food and Nutrition Board. Value shown is the highest RDA for each nutrient, in the year indicated for each revision.

‡ The Dietary Reference Intakes (DRI) are the most recent set of dietary recommendations established by the Food and Nutrition Board of the Institute of Medicine, 1997–2001. They replace previous RDAs, and may be the basis for eventually updating the RDIs. The value shown here is the highest DRI for each nutrient.

§ Historical vitamin E conversion factors were amended in the DRI report, so that 15 mg is defined as the equivalent of 22 IU of natural vitamin E or 33 IU of synthetic vitamin E.

It is recommended that women of childbearing age obtain 400 mcg of synthetic folic acid from fortified breakfast cereals or dietary supplements, in addition to dietary folate.

** It is recommended that people over 50 meet the B-12 recommendation through fortified foods or supplements, to improve bioavailability.

Table 1.2 Minerals: Comparisons Over Time, 1968 to Present

VITAMIN	RDI*	1968 RDA†	1974 RDA†	1980 RDA†	1989 RDA†	DRIs‡
Calcium	1000 mg	1300 mg	1200 mg	1200 mg	1200 mg	1300 mg
Phosphorus	1000 mg	1300 mg	1200 mg	1200 mg	1200 mg	1250 mg
Iron	18 mg	18 mg	18 mg	18 mg	15 mg	18 mg
Iodine	150 mcg	150 mcg	150 mcg	150 mcg	150 mcg	150 mcg
Magnesium	400 mg	400 mg	400 mg	400 mg	400 mg	420 mg
Zinc	15 mg	10–15 mg	15 mg	15 mg	15 mg	11 mg
Selenium	70 mcg	--	--	--	70 mcg	55 mcg
Copper	2 mg	--	--	2–3 mg	1.5–3 mg	0.9 mg
Manganese	2 mg	--	2.5–7 mg	2.5–5 mg	2–5 mg	2.3 mg
Chromium	120 mcg	--	--	50–200 mcg	50–200 mcg	35 mcg
Molybdenum	75 mcg	--	45–500 mcg	150–500 mcg	75–250 mcg	45 mcg

* The Reference Daily Intake (RDI) is the value established by the Food and Drug Administration (FDA) for use in nutrition labeling. It was based initially on the highest 1968 Recommended Dietary Allowance (RDA) for each nutrient, to assure that needs were met for all age groups.

† The RDAs were established and periodically revised by the Food and Nutrition Board. Value shown is the highest RDA for each nutrient, in the year indicated for each revision.

‡ The Dietary Reference Intakes (DRI) are the most recent set of dietary recommendations established by the Food and Nutrition Board of the Institute of Medicine, 1997–2001. They replace previous RDAs, and may be the basis for eventually updating the RDIs. The value shown here is the highest DRI for each nutrient.

Figure 1.1 Making Sense of the Mess

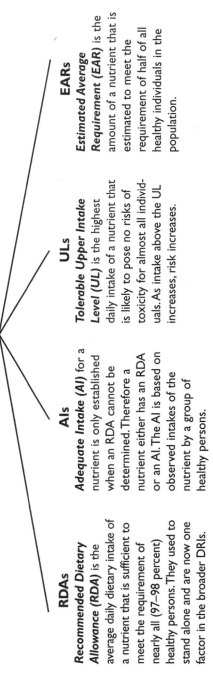

DRIs

Dietary Reference Intake (DRI) is an umbrella group that includes the RDAs, AIs (Adequate Intakes), EARs (Estimated Average Requirements) and ULs (Tolerable Upper Intakes).

RDAs

Recommended Dietary Allowance (RDA) is the average daily dietary intake of a nutrient that is sufficient to meet the requirement of nearly all (97–98 percent) healthy persons. They used to stand alone and are now one factor in the broader DRIs.

AIs

Adequate Intake (AI) for a nutrient is only established when an RDA cannot be determined. Therefore a nutrient either has an RDA or an AI. The AI is based on observed intakes of the nutrient by a group of healthy persons.

ULs

Tolerable Upper Intake Level (UL) is the highest daily intake of a nutrient that is likely to pose no risks of toxicity for almost all individuals. As intake above the UL increases, risk increases.

EARs

Estimated Average Requirement (EAR) is the amount of a nutrient that is estimated to meet the requirement of half of all healthy individuals in the population.

RDIs

Recommended Daily Intake (RDI) takes the place of the old RDAs which appeared on food labels and nutritional information. The old RDAs still exist, but only as a part of the umbrella group DRIs. The RDIs are the guidelines followed by food manufacturers for food labels, and the Percentage Daily Value (%DV) you see on food labels is a measurement of these standards.

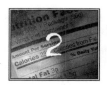

Problems, Problems

While the new DRIs are a vast improvement over the old, stand-alone RDAs, they are still riddled with problems. This chapter will discuss the most glaring of these.

Problem 1: We're All Considered Statistically Average

As the government has been busy morphing the RDAs into the Dietary Reference Intakes (DRIs) in an effort to improve them, we're all still pretty much average. Oh, they're improved, all right, as far as making some adjustments for weight and age. But the biggest problem is the method the government uses to determine what they should be is basically still the same; people are surveyed as to their present diet and the amounts of each nutrient they consume.

Here's how most of their statistical analysis is determined:

In 1956, the National Health and Nutrition Examination Survey (NHANES) was first established in 1956 under the National Health Survey Act to compile statistics and investigate the amount, distribution, and effects of illness and disability in the

United States. Rather than just relying on personal interviews, NHANES conducted clinical tests, measurements, and physical examinations on randomly selected people of all ages, nationalities and economic strata.

During the 1960s, the first of three surveys focused on selected chronic disease of adults aged eighteen to seventy-nine, while later surveys targeted the growth and development of children. The second sample included children aged six to eleven, while the third survey focused on children aged twelve to seventeen. All three surveys had an approximate sample size of 7,500 individuals.

In 1970, a special task force recommended that a continuing surveillance system include studying the link between nutrition, health and disease. They recommended this be done by not just clinical observation and professional assessment but to include recording of eating habits and patterns. Thus, the National Nutrition Surveillance System was combined with the National Health Examination Survey to form the National Health and Nutrition Examination Survey (NHANES).

Although the NHANES studies I and II provided extensive information about the health and nutritional status of the general U.S. population, they did not study individual ethnic groups. So, from 1982 to 1984, NHANES focused on producing estimates of health and nutritional status for the three largest Hispanic subgroups in the United States: Mexican Americans, Cuban Americans, and Puerto Ricans.

NHANES III, conducted between 1988 and 1994, included about forty thousand people selected from households in eighty-one counties across the United States. While including samples of the overall population, by design 30 percent of the participants were black Americans and Mexican Americans. NHANES III was also the first survey to include infants as young as two months of age and to include adults with no upper age limit.

No doubt, the past surveys have produced important results. For example: NHANES showed that low iron levels were a serious problem. As a result, we now have grain and cereals fortified with iron to correct this deficiency.

Past surveys also showed the need for folate to eliminate another deficiency and prevent birth defects. Also, in the 1960s, NHANES led public health officials to sound the alarm about the link between high cholesterol levels and the risk of heart disease.

It was NHANES that gave us the first clear-cut evidence that Americans had too much lead in their blood.

As the food we eat changes—including a wide range of low-fat and light foods—NHANES helps monitor whether these new foods and dietary changes actually are in the best interest of our health. NHANES has turned up important information about the extent of hepatitis B infections and led to the recommendation that all infants and children be vaccinated against it.

The latest NHANES research has already produced some other important conclusions. Specifically, they discovered that about 13 percent of children ages six to eleven are overweight, an increase of 2 percent since 1994. Their older siblings are also getting fatter with the number of overweight subjects ages twelve to nineteen increasing 11 to 14 percent in the same period.

Beginning in 1999, NHANES began a new, continuous, annual survey that can be linked to related Federal Government surveys of the general U.S. population including the USDA Continuing Survey of Food Intakes by Individuals (CSFII), and the Medicare and National Death Index records to help study disease trends.

While in the past, researchers had to wait as long as ten years before gaining access to data based on the entire six-year study to make even the broadest statistical estimates, researchers hope sophisticated sampling techniques and computerization will give them quicker "snapshots" of the nation's health. The number of people examined in a twelve-month period will be about the same as in previous NHANES, about five thousand.

As in the previous NHANES people are screened using random sample selection techniques. This is followed by detailed household interviews. Sample persons are invited to receive physical examinations and health and dietary interviews in mobile examination centers (MECs). Home examinations are given to people unable to come to the MEC for the full examination.

So as impressive as the accomplishment of NHANES might seem, results are based on samples, and averages, meaning, again, we all come out average. Further, the resulting RDA/DRIs don't reflect how much of a given nutrient is needed. Instead, it is a measure of how much the average Joe and Joanne consume. As a result, over time, several nutrient RDAs have been reduced not because of scientific breakthroughs, but as a reflection of changes in the average American diet.

Also, studies on population groups like these can't take into account lifestyle or genetic factors. They often rely on people self-reporting their own dietary habits (assuming they're 100 percent truthful). Often such surveys reflect only short-term eating habits. The fact that every person is an individual with different needs is simply not taken into account. While it's true that everyone needs the same minerals and the same vitamins, as individuals in different circumstances, we need them in differing quantities. In addition, a person's requirements can change dramatically in different circumstances and at different times of life since there are a number of factors effecting the nutritional status of an individual like stress, food allergy, and pregnancy to name a few.

The fact is this system doesn't take into account that we, as individuals, have a unique makeup and experiences. Or, as I recently saw on a bumper sticker, "I'm unique. And so is everyone else."

Problem 1A: Racial Disparities

Ethnic and racial groups have difference nutritional habits, needs and deficiencies. The "one-size-fits-all" approach in the U.S. government's nutritional standards barely addresses the health needs and traditional food customs of African Americans and other racial minorities. Specifically, as the Physicians Committee for Responsible Medicine points out, African Americans have much more lactose intolerance, hypertension, diabetes, cancer, and obesity. Let's look at each of these special needs and concerns:

Lactose intolerance. The guidelines recommend consuming at least two to three servings of dairy products daily, despite the fact that about 70 percent of African Americans are lactose intolerant (compared with only 25 percent of whites) and may suffer from cramping, diarrhea, and bloating after eating dairy products. (Research done as far back as the mid-1960s documents this.) Further, the current guidelines and the related Food Guide Pyramid do not recommend calcium-rich nondairy foods—collard greens, broccoli, kale, beans—which are also low-fat, cholesterol-free, and high in fiber and vitamins. Dairy products, on the other hand, are generally high in fat, cholesterol, sodium, and animal proteins that can hinder calcium absorption.

Hypertension. High blood pressure—which can lead to stroke and congestive heart failure—afflicts about one-third of African Americans, compared to only about one-fourth the general population. Yet, the Dietary Guidelines fail to acknowledge that significantly cutting consumption of fatty foods and dropping meats can help prevent, control, or eliminate hypertension. The guidelines still recommend consumption of meat and dairy products for all Americans.

Diabetes. African Americans have diabetes—a disease that can cause blindness, atherosclerosis, and kidney failure—at a rate 70 percent higher than whites. However, the guidelines recommend consuming fat and animal protein at levels that exacerbate the incidence of diabetes and other diseases.

Cancer. African-American males incur cancer rates 25 percent higher than white males. Prostate cancer, which affects African-American men under 65 at twice the rate of white men, is linked with a diet high in meat and dairy products. But vegetarians and those eating a diet high in rice, soy products, and vegetables have much lower cancer rates. Yet, the Dietary Guidelines do not encourage Americans to replace meat and dairy products with the vegetables, legumes, fruits, and grains that, according to the American Dietetic Association, could reduce the incidence of cancer and other diseases.

Obesity. This remains a serious problem, especially among African-American women. Obesity engenders very serious health problems, including diabetes, stroke, coronary artery disease, kidney disorders, hypertension, and childbirth complications. Studies have shown that individuals on a diet rich in plant foods and low in fat are much less likely to be obese. But the guidelines push meat and dairy products and only recommend a modest reduction in fat—to 30 percent of total calories, rather than a much healthier 10 percent.

Problem 2: Playing with Numbers

To try to cover as many people as possible, the government does massage the numbers a bit. For vitamins and minerals, the recommended amounts are adjusted upward to cover the greatest number of people. To the government's way of thinking, since deficiencies of 30 percent can cause problems while excesses of 300 to 400 percent are generally safe, increasing the RDA by two "standard deviations"—a statistical term—poses little danger. Oh, there are the results of clinical studies added to the mix, but the basic methodology is the same.

Although caloric RDA is determined in the same way, it is not adjusted up or down. To their credit, the USDA recognizes there are problems associated with inadequate caloric intake—such as anorexia—and excess caloric intake, which can lead to obesity. Big surprise, right?

Problem 3: Not Enough Variables

Here's another weakness with the RDAs. In theory, the RDA should allow you to remain free of certain diseases if you consume the minimum. But the effects of lifestyle, local pollution, occupational stress, heredity, climate (sunlight helps make vitamin D), individual biochemistry, among other things, are not—and maybe cannot be—taken into consideration.

The truth is, most of us don't fit into the definition of the average person defined by the RDAs. For example, most adult women don't meet the RDAs for, calcium, magnesium, vitamin B, vitamin E and zinc; likewise, most adult men don't meet the RDAs for magnesium and zinc.

Problem 4: Not Everyone Agrees with Them

As it turns out, not everyone agrees with the new standards. Take, for example, the DRIs for the B vitamins. Based on their nutritional surveys, several of the old standard RDAs were lowered in 1989. When the new DRIs for B vitamins were released in 1998, while many of the B vitamins recommendations were raised slightly—including folic acid to 400 mcg—many nutritionists and researchers thought higher amounts of all the Bs, especially of folic acid, would improve people's health.

Moreover, in 1995, the *New England Journal of Medicine* reported people with high blood levels of a substance called homocysteine were much more likely to have clogged arteries, increasing the likelihood of a heart attack. In their study, the researchers found two-thirds of the people with dangerously high homocysteine had inadequate levels of the three vital Bs. In fact, their study showed the higher levels of three Bs—folic acid, pyridoxine, and cobalamin—helped break down and lower levels of homocysteine and people with the highest B levels cut their risk of a heart attack in half. I don't think you can't find these sorts of things with population studies.

There are those in the USDA that admit other weaknesses in the DRIs. In a presentation she gave in April 1998, Janet King of the Western Human Nutrition Research Center listed four specific problems:

• Only one nutrient was considered at a time.
• Requirements were determined for a single, specified function.
• Recommendations were based primarily on short-term studies.
• DRIs requires translation for consumers.

As for point number one, researchers know nutrients don't act on the body alone. There's a synergy, if you will, between them. Sometimes an excess of one nutrient has a negative effect on others. Sometimes they're more effective in the presence of different nutrients.

As for King's third point, most of the studies used to determine the standards were either "snapshots" or typically conducted for six to nine months—which is only about 1 percent of the average human life span. Nutritional studies with animals have shown that the amounts of some nutrients sufficient to provide health and the prevention of a deficiency disease for short periods of time may be totally inadequate to maintain the health of the animal over its entire lifespan.

Problem 5: What's in a Name?

King's fourth point is very important. The documentation covering the RDAs and DRIs cover multiple volumes and thousands of pages. I'm not so sure that nutritionists and other scientists don't look forward to cuddling up with one of these dry texts any more than you or I would. While the information is important, for the uninitiated it reads like scientific mumbo jumbo.

By now you probably are thoroughly confused, with confusing abbreviations like *RDA*, *RDI*, and *DRI* coming out of your *EARs*. That is part of the problem. Quick! What's the difference between an RDA and an RDI? That's what I thought. They're too perplexing for the average person.

While RDA, RDI and DRI, seem to run together, what they stand for isn't any clearer. I'm willing to bet if you asked a group of people what RDA stands for, many would say the *R* is for *required*, instead of *recommended*. (Personally, I think with the importance of nutrition to our well-being, *required* would be a much better term.)

Also, a large group of people would misidentify the *D* as *daily* and not *dietary*. And why allowance? To my way of thinking, an allowance is something you give to your kids (who probably spend a large chunk of it on junk food).

I think the term *DRI* is even worse. While the first word *Dietary* is fine, I think *Reference Intake* for *RI* makes most people want to cover their ears and shout "La, La-La, La, La."

When deciding what to eat, the average conscientious person wants to know whether a particular food is good for them. I doubt if anyone ever says, "Hmmm. This broccoli stalk really helps fulfill my Reference Intake." Yeah . . . right.

If these nutritional standards are intended to guide us to nutritional well-being, why give them high-falutin' names?

Problem 6: Unrealistic Standards

For optimum health from certain nutrients, the standards are virtually impossible to achieve just from eating. Take the case of vitamin E. The RDA for vitamin E is 30 International Units (IU). Two good sources of vitamin E are peanuts and brown rice. In order to get the RDA for vitamin E from these foods you would need to eat ten ounces of peanuts at 1,050 calories or over two pounds of brown rice at 1,575 calories.

Even worse, research shows to take advantage of the many health protective benefits of vitamin E, you should be getting between 200 and 400 IU daily. How much food does it take to get to that level? Well, you'd have to eat 40 cups of peanuts or 130 cups of brown rice. Take your choice? The peanuts would add 33,600 calories. The rice? 91,000 calories.

Problem 7: Lack of Worldwide Consistency

The RDAs/DRIs are not just some quirk of the U.S.A. For years the U.S. RDA was generally accepted throughout the world with more than forty countries and health organizations publishing similar—but not exact—standards. The Canadian equivalent, the Recommended Nutrient Intakes (RNI), is virtually the same and the DRIs are actually a joint project between the U.S. and Canada.

But while standards throughout the world are similar, there are some noticeable differences. For example, the RDA for vitamin A in Switzerland and Columbia is 50 percent higher than in the United States and Canada. Are these differences based solely on ethnic differences? Do people in Hispanic Columbia—a tropical country—and northern European Switzerland—which is not the least bit tropical—have greater similarities in their nutritional needs, than say, North Americans? I wouldn't think so.

Problem 8: What about Future Breakthroughs?

Then there's the issue of cutting-edge, scientific breakthroughs. It seems nearly every week, we hear of research findings that cast a new, favorable light on a nutrient, or discover previous findings aren't quite so grand as originally thought. Take the case of vitamin E. Not so long ago, it was thought to be nonessential. Today, it's trumpeted as a key to fighting off many illnesses and aging. It will take quite a while for new information to be incorporated into the DRIs not just because changes have to go up the "chain of command," but because there is a natural tendency by the government to take things very slowly until "all the facts are in."

But as in the case of vitamin E, it makes you wonder. How many other "nonessential" nutrients such as the flavonoids, carotenoids, minerals and trace minerals will turn out to be essential? How long will it be before we see them in the government standards? Also, our diets probably already contain many essential nutrients yet undiscovered.

What about the nutrients the RDAs don't mention at all? We'll discuss those further in a later chapter.

Problem 9: No One Can Predict the Future

Researchers admit scientific knowledge of nutritional requirements is far from complete: that the requirements for many nutrients have not been established; that several essential nutrients have only recently been discovered; and that in all likelihood other nutrients will be found to be essential in years to come. So what do they recommend in the meantime? Eat a varied diet, and do not depend on pills or processed foods artificially stoked with known micronutrients.

Problem 10: One Size Fits All, and It's Small

Here's another weakness with the standards. The RDAs have long reflected the amounts of selected nutrients considered adequate to meet the known nutrient needs of healthy people.

There are two key words here: *healthy* and *adequate*. Here's where the equality of all people—although *inequality* is probably more accurate—comes into play. For example, according to the most recent guidelines, an eleven-year-old boy—regardless of his size—needs the same amount of vitamin E as a man in his fifties. Likewise, a twenty-five-year-old woman needs the same amount of vitamin C (60 mg) as a fifty-five-year-old woman *or* man.

When an RDA amount does vary based on gender or age, it's usually not by much. The guidelines for protein provide a good example. Here, the RDA for a female between the ages of eleven and fourteen is 46 grams of protein. Once that same female reaches fifteen, she needs only 44 grams, a 4 percent decrease. Incidentally, the amount goes back up to 46 grams when the girl reaches the age of nineteen.

Throughout the RDA list of nutrients—which includes all the vitamins and many minerals, protein and a few other substances—you find the same pattern. Even though age and weight are now factored in to the RDAs to some degree, for the most part, one size still fits all, regardless of race, creed or national origin.

I don't buy it. Just as every individual is endowed with a unique set of genes and has a unique history of physical, biochemical, nutritional and emotional experiences, so is the measure of optimal health is probably unique for each of us.

It's true that most of us don't know people suffering from scurvy (lack of vitamin C) or beriberi—since even most people with the worst eating habits manage to avoid these diseases. However, it's no secret that for the majority of the U.S. population the diet is lacking in essential nutrients. In fact, many studies show that half of all Americans older than sixty years are deficient in vitamins A, C, and E, even by the minimum standard RDA. And while they might not get scurvy, rickets (lack of vitamin D) or beriberi (from a thiamin deficiency), they do suffer from a myriad of other diseases such as cancer, cardiovascular problems and diabetes.

Remember, the minimum daily requirement refers to the absolute minimum amount you need of the vitamin, a bare-bones amount that will keep you from suffering from a vitamin deficiency. As a result, miraculously, we never hear of people suffering from deficiency diseases because somewhere in that candy bar, hot dog, French fries and milk shake, they've managed to digest at least the minimum nutrient requirement. But at what cost?

Optimal means "the best we can be." Personally, I'd rather opt for optimum health, and, I suspect you do too.

Problem 11: Predicting Average Requirements

As I've written, RDAs don't point out how much of a specific nutrient you need on a daily basis, but rather the "average" minimum recommended to maintain body processes and minimize deficiency symptoms.

The USDA and NAS admit that while the average requirement for each nutrient is probably closest to most people's need. If all persons were to stick to the average, we would probably have a situation where half the population would develop deficiencies of some sort. They warn, though, that a person should not take more than the average recommended nutrient, as this may lead to going above "upper safe" level, where some nutrients can be toxic.

While they do say the individuality of requirements is the key, they admit their tables provide only examples as to what the average nutrient intake should be. According to the definitions of "safe and adequate" ranges, "safe" means "not too high" and "adequate" means "not too low."

Problem 12: Shifting Standards

Before you call me a hypocrite, let me explain something. I know I just finished telling you the DRI standards don't change rapidly enough to reflect new and helpful nutrient information. And now, I'm going to criticize the NAS and USDA for making changes. I'm specifically referring to the NAS *Dietary Reference Intakes for Energy, Carbohydrate, Fiber, Fat, Fatty Acids, Cholesterol, Protein, and Amino Acids*, published in September 2002.

Prior to the publication of these new guidelines, I offered the following criticisms, and for good reason; the old standards, if followed, could have a huge impact on a person's health.

The NAS is to be congratulated for "getting it mostly right" with the new guidelines, but the differences from the old RDAs are so important they should be shouted from the rooftops and not buried in a nine hundred-page scientific report.

Now, of course I had a good part of this book written before the NAS released the new guidelines, so I had to change a few things. It should be helpful to get an idea of how well the NAS has done so far, and to see how far it has yet to go. First, I'll report my pre-September 2002 concerns about the "old" standards, followed by what the NAS is now saying (in quotes).

Regarding energy RDAs. Prior to seeing the new NAS standards released in September 2002 I wrote the following: *It's common sense that in order for a person to maintain their body weight, the amount of food energy they take in must equal the energy expended. The average energy consumption is aimed at setting a standard for people to work from and gives an example of how many calories are reasonable for each group. It's interesting that an output side of the energy balance equation, in other words how much energy people should expend, has not been established.*

In September 2002, the NAS reported, "To maintain cardiovascular health at a maximal level, regardless of weight, adults and children also should spend a total of at least one hour each day in moderately intense physical activity, which is double the daily goal set by the 1996 Surgeon General's report."

The report goes on to stress the importance of balancing diet with exercise, recommending total calories to be consumed by individuals of a given height, weight, and gender for each of four different levels of physical activity.

"For example," says the NAS, "a thirty-year-old woman who is 5 feet 5 inches tall and weighs 111 to 150 pounds should consume between 1,800 and 2,000 calories daily if she lives a sedentary lifestyle. However, if she is a very active person, her recommended total caloric intake increases to 2,500 to 2,800 calories per day. If her lifestyle fits the moderately active category as defined in the report, which is the minimum level of activity to decrease risk of chronic disease, she should eat between 2,200 and 2,500 calories daily. Using grams for the recommended ranges of intake, she should consume 55 to 97 grams of fat and 285 to 375 grams of carbohydrates per day."

The new one-hour-a-day-total exercise goal stems from studies on how much energy is expended on average each day by individuals who maintain a healthy weight. "Energy expenditure is cumulative, including both low-intensity activities of daily life, such as stair climbing and housecleaning, and more vigorous exercise like swimming and cycling. Someone in a largely sedentary occupation can achieve the new exercise goal by engaging in a moderate-intensity activity, such as walking at four miles per hour, for a total of sixty minutes every day. They can also engage in a high-intensity activity, such as jogging for twenty to thirty minutes four to seven days per week."

While the NAS should be applauded for adding these important new guidelines, my earlier criticism still stands; these standards are based on "averages" derived from "population studies."

Regarding protein RDAs. Prior to seeing the new NAS standards released in September 2002, I wrote the following: *Protein recommendations are mainly based on the individual's body weight. The protein RDA is high, to cover most person's needs. The average requirement for protein is 0.6 grams per kilogram of body weight; the RDA is 0.8 grams. This standard is said to meet 97.5 percent of the population's needs.*

In September 2002, the NAS reported, "Protein intake recommendations are the same." However, the NAS goes on to say, "The report establishes age-based requirements for the first time for all nine of the essential amino acids found in dietary protein. Values are included for pregnant women, infants, and children based on their special needs.

Using new data, the report reaffirms previously established recommended levels of protein intake, which is 0.8 grams per kilogram of body weight for adults. Recommended intake of protein during pregnancy also is increased. Because data on the potential for high-protein diets to produce chronic or other diseases are often conflicting or inadequate, tolerable upper intake levels for consumption could not be determined for protein or for the individual amino acids.

However, given the lack of data on overconsumption for some of these amino acids and protein, caution is warranted in consuming levels significantly above those normally found in foods."

Regarding RDA for carbohydrate and fat. Prior to seeing the new NAS standards released in September 2002, I wrote the following: *The amount of protein recommended represents a small percentage of a person's energy allowance, with the remainder acquired from carbohydrates and fats. The general guideline for carbohydrate and fat is that more than half of daily energy should come from carbohydrates, with no more than one third from fat. However, there are no specific recommendations for either. In this day and age with so much emphasis—and misinformation—about good and bad fat, and the need for carbohydrates, these issues are too important to be ignored.*

In September 2002, the NAS reported, "Because carbohydrates, fat, and protein all serve as energy sources and can substitute for one another to some extent to meet caloric needs, the recommended ranges for consuming these nutrients should be useful and flexible for dietary planning.

"Earlier guidelines called for diets with 50 percent or more of carbohydrates and 30 percent or less of fat." (Again, protein intake recommendations are the same.)

"The new acceptable ranges for children are similar to those for adults, except that infants and younger children need a slightly higher proportion of fat—25 percent to 40 percent of their caloric intake, said the panel that wrote the report.

"'We established ranges for fat, carbohydrates, and protein because they must be considered together,'" said panel chair Joanne Lupton, professor of nutrition at Texas A&M University. "'Studies show that when people eat very low levels of fat combined with very high levels of carbohydrates, high-density lipoprotein concentration, or good cholesterol, decreases. Conversely, high-fat diets can lead to obesity and its complications if caloric intake is increased as well, which is often the case. We believe these ranges will help people make healthy and more realistic choices based on their own food preferences.'"

To their credit, the NAS does make a bold stand in their September 2002 report regarding "sweets." The report says that while both children and adults should consume at least 130 grams of carbohydrates each day, "the newly set RDA is based on the minimum amount of carbohydrates needed to produce enough glucose for the brain to function, and most people regularly consume far more." The report recommends added sugars should not comprise more than 25 percent of total calories consumed. "Distinguished from natural sugars, such as lactose found in milk and fructose found in fruits, added sugars are those incorporated into foods and beverages during production," says the NAS. "Major sources [of added sugar] include candy, soft drinks, fruit drinks, pastries, and other sweets. The suggested maximum level stems from the evidence that people whose diets are high in added sugars have lower intakes of essential nutrients." More on fat and carbohydrates in a later chapter.

Regarding fiber. Prior to seeing the new NAS standards released in September 2002, I wrote the following: *There is no recommendation for fiber; however, it is recommended that sufficient fiber be obtained from fruits, vegetables, legumes, and whole-grain products (all of which also provide vitamins, minerals and water). A lack of fiber in the diet can cause a myriad of health problems and is too important for the USDA and NAS to give only a token nod.*

In September 2002, the NAS reported: "The report contains the first recommended intake levels for fiber from the Food and Nutrition Board. The fiber recommendations are based on studies that show an increased risk for heart disease when diets low in fiber are consumed. Although there is some evidence to suggest that fiber in the diet may also help to prevent colon cancer and promote weight control, the data are inconclusive at this point.

"The recommended daily intake for total fiber for adults fifty years and younger is set at 38 grams for men and 25 grams for women, while for men and women over fifty it is 30 and 21 grams per day, respectively, due to decreased consumption of food."

The report also provides recommended intakes for children and teenagers: "Many new food products are marketed as containing fiber, but the lack of a uniform definition of fiber for regulatory purposes casts doubts on the usefulness of some content claims."

Therefore, the report provides a specific definition of what should be called fiber in food. It defines "total fiber" as the combination of "dietary" and "functional" fiber.

"Dietary fiber is the edible, nondigestible component of carbohydrates and lignin naturally found in plant food." (Foods with dietary fiber include cereal bran, flaked corn cereal, sweet potatoes, legumes, and onions.)

"Functional fiber refers to those fiber sources that are shown to have similar health benefits as dietary fiber, but are isolated or extracted from natural sources or are synthetic." (An example would be pectin extracted from citrus peel and used as a gel that is the basis for jams and jellies.)

The definition of functional fiber excludes fiber-like products, whether extracted or synthesized, that cannot be shown to have proven health benefits. "It is hoped that regulatory bodies in both the United States and Canada will work toward adopting these definitions," says the NAS.

Problem 13: What's Not Included

There are plenty of substances found in our foods not included in the RDAs and DRIs. We'll cover those in a later chapter; however, there is one omission I'd like to mention here.

Lately, you often see people, especially women—even those dressed in business attire—walking down the street slurping on a water bottle. This is understandable since it's been drummed into people that they need at least eight 8-ounce glasses of liquids a day (with greater needs depending on a person's size and level of activity). While the USDA and NAS recognize water consumption is an area neglected by most individuals, they fail to consider climatic, exercise and age-related needs.

To complicate things even further, a new concern has recently arisen: Do people really need this much water? And if so, what are the best pure sources? We'll cover water in a later chapter.

Problem 14: Is "Upper Safe" High Enough?

The Upper Safe Limits indicates an amount of a nutrient that appears safe for most healthy people. However, the standards go on to say some people might experience toxicity symptoms at these levels and recommend that more "diligent" individuals seek advice regarding their own personal needs relating to their height, weight and their daily amount of energy expenditure. Apparently, they think the "diligent" are the exception and not the rule.

In most cases, the Upper Safe Limits are very conservative. While it appears the USDA and NAS would rather err on the side of caution, it's also possible we might not be getting the most benefit from nutrients because of a false fear of toxicity.

For example, in a recent article in the *International Journal of Basic and Applied Nutritional Sciences*, Katherine Milton, a Professor of Environmental Science at the University of California, studied the eating habits of primates in the Panamanian Nature Reserve. She found the following: A 15-pound wild monkey consumes 600 mg of vitamin C per day, ten times more than the daily recommendation for humans. The monkeys consumed 4,571 mg of calcium per day, nearly twice as much as the Upper Safe Limit for humans. The monkeys ate 6,419 mg of potassium per day. Typically, humans eat only between one-third and one-half of that amount.

Now granted, most of us don't spend our days expending our energy swinging from vines, and of course, it's sometimes faulty to compare the results of studies on animals with humans. Still, some of the scientific research conducted by the NAS panels incorporate findings not just on animals, but also blood samples from humans, so Milton's research just might show our standards are more cautious than necessary.

Problem 15: Consumer Indifference

Here's perhaps the biggest weakness in the RDAs and DRIs; most people just don't follow them. What good are standards if most people ignore the advice? How many people actually eat an adequate, balanced diet if not every day, at least most days? I'm talking about a diet with plenty of vitamins, fiber and minerals including fresh fruits and vegetables, whole-grain breads and cereals, low-fat dairy products, skinless poultry, fish, and lean meats (low in saturated fat and cholesterol). When I say whole-grain bread, I don't mean the lightweight spongy stuff found in most grocery stores; I mean the thick heavy stuff you actually have to chew. And whole-grain cereals? Don't ask.

A few years ago, the USDA conducted a survey of over twenty-one thousand people's minimum daily requirements (and remember the minimums are barely adequate.) For example, while the RDA for vitamin C for most people is only 60 mg (which you can achieve by drinking a single glass of orange juice), not one person, *not a one—* was getting that much vitamin C. Never mind that even higher levels of vitamin C can protect you from a myriad of diseases.

I don't know why people don't get enough vitamin C. Maybe it is because people by and large are lackadaisical, or maybe it's because they figure if it's for sale, it must be good for us (especially with so many food product sporting names including words like *nature*, *down-home* and even *Grandma's*).

Maybe they think standards impinge on their right to gorge themselves on anything they like. Or, maybe, and I tend to favor this one, the standards are just too complicated and are presented in a way that just doesn't inspire people to change their eating habits.

Ask yourself (and although this is not a quiz, your body will be giving you a grade), how often do you eat fat-laden, salty fast food? Do you eat fresh fruit on a daily basis, or is biannually a better measure? Are you more familiar with a vending machine than a food processor? Do you far exceed the RDA for chocolate candy bars? Numerous studies show fewer than 30 percent of people eat five fresh fruits and vegetables a day with 20 percent admitting they don't eat *any* fruits or vegetables at all.

Let's face the facts—despite thousands and thousands of dry written pages supporting the new DRIs, there is one underlying principal determining our nutritional health: It's not how much you eat. It's *what* you eat.

While the DRIs are a vast improvement over the RDAs, chances are people are not going to follow them. "The truth is that people are still confused about how their dietary behavior contributes to health risk," says Dr. Paula A. Quatromoni, co-author of a study in published in the September 2002 issue of the *Journal of the American Dietetic Association*. Quatromoni continues, "And people are frustrated with the controversy that exists, with arguments even among nutrition experts as to whether it's the amount of fat or the type of fat that matters most; whether high-carbohydrate diets are good for you; whether low-fat diets are appropriate either."

While the study, conducted by the Boston University School of Public Health in Massachusetts, focuses on women (who—men let's be honest—usually take better care of themselves than men), their conclusions apply to both genders.

What the researchers set out to find was, can current dietary patterns among women of normal weight predict whether they will become overweight? After studying 737 non-overweight women over a twelve-year period, the researchers found women who are not overweight but who indulge in a high-fat, high-sugar diet filled with empty calories are most likely to become overweight in later years. Specifically, they discovered 29 percent of the women in the study became overweight.

Based on this, Quatromoni determined that women who are "junk-food junkies" are 40 percent more likely to become overweight than those who eat a heart-healthy diet rich in fruits and vegetables and low-fat, high-fiber foods. Those women whose weight fluctuated due to yo-yo dieting had a slightly higher risk of being overweight. But there's another factor that has had a profound influence on the government's nutritional recommendations, as you'll see in the next chapter.

Listing all the RDA and DRI data would leave most people glass-eyed, so I decided to include a few tables that provide some of the more important data.

Table 2.1 Protein and Fat-Soluble Vitamins: Recommendations by Age

	Age	Energy kcal	Protein grams*	Vitamin A IU mcg*		Vitamin D IU mcg*		Vitamin E IU mg*		Vitamin K mcg†
Children	4–6	1,800	3.0/24	2,500	500	400	5	9	7	20
	7–10	2,000	3.6/28	3,300	500	400	5	10	7	30
Males	15–18	3,000	5.4/59	5,000	1,000	400	5	15	10	65
	19–24	2,900	5.4/58	5,000	1,000	400	5	15	10	70
	25–50	2,700	5.6/63	5,000	1,000	400	5	15	10	80
	50+	2,400	5.6/63	5,000	1,000	800	10	15	10	80
Females	15–18	2,100	4.8/44	4,000	1,000	400	5	12	8	55
	19–24	2,100	4.6/46	4,000	800	400	5	12	8	60
	25–50	2,100	4.6/50	4,000	800	400	5	12	8	65
	50+	1,800	4.6/50	4,000	800	800	10	12	8	65

* The first figure refers to the old RDA listing while the second figure refers to the new DRI listing.
† Previous guidelines did not include an RDA for vitamin K.
Source: USDA and the Council for Responsible Nutrition

Table 2.2 Water-Soluble Vitamins: Recommendations by Age

	Age	Vitamin C mg*	Folic Acid mcg*	Niacin mg*	Riboflavin mg*	Thiamin mg*	Vitamin B6 mg*	Vitamin B12 mcg*
Children	4–6	40/45	200/75	12	1.1	0.9	09/1.1	1.5/1.0
	7–10	40/45	300/100	16/13	1.2	1.2/1.0	1.2	2.0/1.4
Males	15–18	45/60	400/200	20	1.8	1.5	2	3.0/2.0
	19–24	45/60	400/200	20/19	1.8/1.7	1.5	2	3.0/2.0
	25–50	45/60	400/200	19/18	1.6/1.7	1.4/1.5	2	3.0/2.0
	50+	45/60	400/200	16/15	1.5/1.4	1.2	2	3.0/2.0
Females	15–18	45/60	400/180	15/14	1.4/1.3	1.1	2.0/1.5	3.0/2.0
	19–24	45/60	400/180	15/14	1.4/1.3	1.1	2.0/1.6	3.0/2.0
	25–50	45/60	400/180	15/13	1.2/1.3	1.0/1.1	2.0/1.6	3.0/2.0
	50+	45/60	400/180	13/12	1.1/1.2	1	2.0/1.6	3.0/2.0

* The first figure refers to the old RDA listing while the second figure refers to the new DRI listing.

† Previous guidelines did not include an RDA.

Source: USDA and the Council for Responsible Nutrition

Table 2.3 Minerals: Recommendations by Age

Age	Calcium mg	Phosphorus mg	Iodine mcg	Iron mg	Magnesium mg	Zinc mg	Selenium mcg†	Flouride mg†
Children 4–6	800	800/500	80/90	10	200/130	10	20	1.1
7–10	800	800	110/120	10	250	10	30	3.2
Males 15–18	800/1,000	1,200/1,250	150	10	400/410	15	50	3.8
19–24	800/1,000	800/700	140/150	10	350/400	15	70	3.8
25–50	800/1,000	800/700	130/150	10	350/420	15	70	3.8
50+	800/1,000	200–400	110/150	10	350/420	15	70	2.9
Females 15–18	1200/1,300	1,200/1,250	115/150	18/15	300/360	15/12	50	3.1
19–24	800/1,000	800/700	100/150	18/15	300/310	15/12	55	3.1
25–50	800/1,000	800/700	100/150	18/15	300/320	15/12	55	3.1
50+	800/1,000	800/700	80/150	10	300/320	15/12	55	3.1

* The first figure refers to the old RDA listing while the second figure refers to the new DRI listing.

† Previous guidelines did not include an RDA.

Source: USDA and the Council for Responsible Nutrition

Table 2.4 Comparisons of RDIs, DRIs, and ULs for Vitamins

VITAMIN	Current RDI*	New DRI†	UL‡
Vitamin A	5000 IU	3000 IU	10000 IU
Vitamin C	60 mg	90 mg	2000 mg
Vitamin D	10 mcg	15 mcg	50 mcg
Vitamin E	20 mg	15 mg	1000 mg
Vitamin K	80 mcg	120 mcg	ND
Thiamin	1.5 mg	1.2 mg	ND
Riboflavin	1.7 mg	1.3 mg	ND
Niacin	20 mg	16 mg	35 mg
Vitamin B6	2 mg	1.7 mg	100 mg
Folate	400 mcg	400 mcg	1000 mcg
Vitamin B12	6 mcg	2.4 mcg	ND
Biotin	300 mcg	30 mcg	ND
Pantothenic	10 mg	5 mg	ND
Choline	--	550 mg	3500 mg

* The Reference Daily Intake (RDI) is the value established by the Food and Drug Administration (FDA) for use in nutrition labeling. It was based initially on the highest 1968 Recommended Dietary Allowance (RDA) for each nutrient, to assure that needs were met for all age groups.

† The Dietary Reference Intakes (DRI) are the most recent set of dietary recommendations established.

‡ The Upper Limit (UL) is the upper level of intake considered to be safe for use by adults, incorporating a safety factor. In some cases, lower ULs have been established for children.

ND Upper Limit not determined. No adverse effects observed from high intakes of the nutrient.

Source: USDA and the Council for Responsible Nutrition

Table 2.5 Comparisons of RDIs, DRIs, and ULs for Minerals

Mineral	Current RDI*	New DRI†	UL‡
Calcium	1,000 mg	1,300 mg	2,500 mg
Iron	18 mg	18 mg	45 mg
Phosphorus	1,000 mg	1,250 mg	4,000 mg
Iodine	150 mcg	150 mcg	1,100 mcg
Magnesium	400 mg	420 mg	350 mg§
Zinc	15 mg	11 mg	40 mg
Selenium	70 mg	55 mg	400 mg
Copper	2 mg	0.9 mg	10 mg
Manganese	2 mg	2.3 mg	11 mg
Chromium	120 mcg	35 mcg	ND
Molybdenum	75 mcg	45 mcg	2,000 mcg

* The Reference Daily Intake (RDI) is the value established by the Food and Drug Administration (FDA) for use in nutrition labeling. It was based initially on the highest 1968 Recommended Dietary Allowance (RDA) for each nutrient, to assure that needs were met for all age groups.

† The Dietary Reference Intakes (DRI) are the most recent set of dietary recommendations established.

‡ The Upper Limit (UL) is the upper level of intake considered to be safe for use by adults, incorporating a safety factor. In some cases, lower ULs have been established for children.

§ Upper Limit for magnesium applies only to intakes from dietary supplements or pharmaceutical products, not including intakes from food and water.

ND Upper Limit not determined. No adverse effects observed from high intakes of the nutrient.

Source: USDA and the Council for Responsible Nutrition

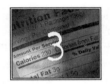

Who's Really Talking?

The next time you're out in public, look at the people on your left and right. Chances are at least one of the three of you is overweight and another one of you is obese—possibly extremely obese.

It should be obvious that in our "Land of Plenty" plenty of us are getting good and fat. According to an October 2002 study from the Centers for Disease Control and Prevention (CDC), one in every three U.S. adults is now obese and nearly two-thirds are overweight.

Just so you know, according to the CDC:

- You are overweight if you have a body mass index of 25 or higher. (For example, a 5-foot, 6-inch person who weighs 160 pounds or more.)
- Obesity is defined as having a BMI of 30 or greater.
- Extreme obesity is defined as having a BMI of 40 or more. This is equal to a 5-foot, 10-inch person weighing 280 pounds or more.

What do these facts have to do with our nutritional guidelines? Plenty. First of all, this data is further proof our nutritional guidelines are wrong, aren't being followed, or aren't working. Second, since a key part of data for the RDA/DRIs is based on "average eating habits," will these obesity statistics skew our needs upward in future reports? This theory might be a stretch, but maybe not.

Health experts, including George L. Blackburn, chairman of nutrition medicine at Harvard Medical School, say the latest obesity findings show we are totally losing the battle to prevent and treat obesity. Especially troubling is the rise in extreme obesity. In the CDC study, the number of adults with extreme obesity rose from 3 percent to nearly 5 percent from 1999 to 2000. This trend concerns public health officials, because adults today are at greater risk for severe health problems, including diabetes, high blood pressure, heart disease and kidney failure.

This is not something that happened overnight, although it is increasing rapidly. Despite spending $34 billion annually on diet products—including diet and low-fat foods, weight-loss supplements and diet programs—the CDC reports the number of overweight adults rose from 56 percent to 65 percent of the population between 1999 to 2000. That's just one year!

While waistlines are expanding across the board, the study shows that some groups are getting fatter faster than others. For example, more than half of black women forty and older are obese, and more than 80 percent are overweight.

The obesity epidemic is not limited to adults. A companion study of children and adolescents, led by Cynthia L. Ogden of the CDC's National Center for Health Statistics, found that in 1999 to 2000, nearly 16 percent of twelve- to nineteen-year-olds were overweight, an increase of nearly 5 percentage points from 1988 to 1994. Among black and Mexican American adolescents, the rise was even greater, jumping 10 percent.

About 7 percent of youngsters two to five were overweight in 1988 to 1994, according to the CDC. But from 1999 to 2000, that number rose to 10 percent. Among those six to eleven, the number of overweight children increased from 11 percent in 1988 to 1994 to 15 percent in 1999 to 2000.

"This is a stunning increase and a really scary thing," said Richard L. Atkinson, president of the American Obesity Association and director of the Medstar Research Institute's obesity research. "The public health costs of this are just really frightening if the disease acts as it has in adults. It certainly portends a grave public health problem."

In an editorial that accompanies the obesity studies appearing in the *Journal of the American Medical Association*, deputy editor Phil B. Fontanarosa writes that "during a time when the amount of research activity, knowledge and interest in obesity among the medical community, as well as the level of public attention to the issues of weight, diet and exercise have never been greater, the epidemic of obesity continues virtually unabated with no sign of reversal."

What might even be worse is that while the richest nation in the world is becoming more and more obese, it is becoming more and more nutritionally starved.

Big Deal, or No Big Deal?

When statistics on the obesity epidemic like these come out, people generally have one of five reactions:

1. Concern and a concerted effort to improve their habits.

2. A belief that the numbers are wrong. "The CDC's report is flaky in its scientific quality, misleading in its presentation to the public and disturbing in its agenda," wrote frequent critic Steve Milloy, an adjunct scholar at the Cato Institute and publisher of JunkScience.com, when a previous CDC obesity report was issued in 2000. Milloy especially dislikes the way the CDC gathers its data; largely via random questionnaires over the telephone. (Not unlike political races: the candidate who's ahead trumpets the results, while the one who's behind pooh-poohs them.)

3. Some people say, "So what's the big deal? We like being well fed." I would normally agree. If you want to be fat, that's your business, except in the end we all pay; when you're overweight you increase the likelihood of serious illness, including diabetes, coronary problems and cancer. For example, type II (adult onset) diabetes is totally preventable. Most people can prevent it by eating less—and not even that much less.

4. Others will say, "The government—especially the CDC—has no business looking at this problem"; or "The CDC should concentrate on communicable diseases."

Milloy is a strong supporter of this point. He writes "There is no doubt that there are many obese individuals in the U.S. Nor is there doubt that obese individuals have greater rates of heart disease, diabetes and other health problems. But while obesity is not a desirable condition for most people, is it really 'a critical public health problem' that needs to be addressed like as an 'infectious disease epidemic'? Should obesity be likened to epidemics of malaria, typhus, cholera, smallpox and the plague? Or is this just a case of 'fat police brutality'?"

5. Then there are others who say people need to take responsibility for themselves—show some self-control.

Maybe some of us are too anxious to turn our ire on the messenger. While no one likes the government as big brother, the fact is whether it comes from the CDC, National Institute of Health, or the Department of Bells and Whistles, it doesn't alter the scary facts. (Again, look to your left and look to your right.) No one is showing up at our front doors and *forcing* us to exercise or lose weight, and I can't imagine they ever will.

This point gets a little sticky. As we should have learned from our nation's romance with—then condemnation of—tobacco, it is possible for part of the government to revile something in one building while subsidizing that same thing in another building. In the case of food, our will power and self-control are severely tested everyday by a powerful and clever industry that aggressively markets to our weaknesses.

Take This Simple Test

We all have to eat, and the competition for our food dollars is fierce. In the year 2000, food companies grossed nearly $900 billion in sales.

The next time you're watching TV and a fast food ad comes on, hold up the RDA/DRI chart from the previous chapter. Now, look at the chart, then look at the juicy burger, succulent fried chicken, or steaming hot pizza. Which would you rather sink your teeth into?

I know—it's not fair. The food industry knows it too. They employ a bunch of marketing whizzes and psychologists, and they use focus groups and reams of consumer studies to get you to buy their products. You have only, well—little 'ol you, and bland statistics from the CDC to combat their marketing campaigns.

It's a tough battle to win. Let's face it—the food tastes good, and the message about healthy eating is very boring. And the food industry usually wins.

Food Glorious Food

The U.S. food industry produces an estimated 3,800 calories a day for every person in the U.S., up from 3,300 calories a day in the 1970s. On average, (sorry—there's the "average" label again) women need about 2,200 calories a day, men need about 2,500. Since most of us are gaining weight, we're obviously eating more than that.

It isn't about only will power. The food industry actively promotes overeating by spending $10 billion a year in direct media advertising. It also spends another $20 billion a year in indirect marketing, including things like toy prizes, sponsorships or sporting events logos on school scoreboards.

That is considerably more money than is spent on health and nutrition education. For example, the campaign for fruits and vegetables spends about $2 million a year on public education.

Over-indulgence is so acceptable today; people think drinking soft drinks all the time is normal, and you're expected to pig out at sporting events. You're constantly told in subtle—and not-so subtle—ways to eat more.

Take portion sizes—it's no coincidence that promoting larger portions started at the same time that obesity rates started to go up. And it's not just fast-food chains; muffins used to be 1 or 2 ounces; now they're 6 or 7. Order pasta or Chinese food, and you're served enough food to feed six people. Then there's the buffets and all-you-can-eat specials.

More Help than Needed

As I've mentioned earlier, the food industry in the U.S. produces nearly double the amount of calories needed by every person.

To make sure its industry or company gets its share, the food industry does whatever it can to persuade people to eat more food, more often, and in larger portions than is healthy. How better to influence what people eat than with official government standards and policies?

When Marion Nestle, Ph.D., M.P.H., worked on the 1988 Surgeon General's *Report on Nutrition and Health*, she found plenty of people willing to help her. She quickly realized their motives weren't all altruistic. Rather, not-so-secret agendas quickly came into play. Nestle—yes, that's her real name—discovered that the food industry plays politics as well as any other industry. And it's not whiffle ball they're playing, but hardball; spikes-up, brush-back hardball.

Nestle, who is now the head of New York University's department of nutrition and food studies, says one particular industry's representatives were constantly in her office pressuring her not to say their product was bad, or that consumption of it should be restricted. When her book, *Food Politics*, came out in 2002 and she criticized this particular industry, they threatened to sue her.

Since I don't want them to sue me, I can't tell you what food industry threatened her. I can give you only clues:

Clue 1: It's white
Clue 2: It's sweet
Clue 3: It's granular

Likewise, other food groups pressured her, including the same one that sued talk show hostess Oprah Winfrey a few years back after she lambasted their product—helping cause its commodity prices to fall to ten-year lows in the days after her comments. This particular organization's product is linked to over-consumption of saturated fat. Again, I can't tell you who they are. I can give you only a clue. (Their main product chews its cud and makes a sound like "moo.")

To get around recommendations to eat less of these two foods (along with other foods whose lobbyists were pressuring Nestle) the government compromised: The 1988 report didn't say eat less products that go "moo," it says "choose lean meat." It also doesn't say eat less white, sweet, granular stuff; it says "choose a diet moderate in" such things.

Dr. Nestle remains undaunted: "Many of the nutritional problems of Americans, not the least of them obesity, can be traced to the food industry's imperative to encourage people to eat more in order to generate sales and increase income."

It starts with breakfast. Let's take the standard (and very popular) fruit rings cereal—it has no fruit, no fiber, and *half* its calories come from sugar. While it's fortified with some vitamins and minerals, it's certainly not fruit, and it's not a health food. In fact, it's probably closer to candy than part of a well-rounded breakfast. Yet, it meets "government standards."

Nestle has her share of critics. In a February 22, 2002 article on FOXNews.com, entitled "New Nutrition Book Choking on Bad Science" Steven Milloy skewered Nestle and her book, *Food Politics*.

Millow wrote, "Despite the folklore developed over the last thirty years, the role of saturated fat in heart disease risk remains uncertain." A recent Harvard University study of more than eighty thousand women, for example, reported no statistical association between saturated fat intake and heart disease. If the folklore were true, such a large study would likely have verified it.

Milloy goes on to accuse Dr. Nestle of encouraging readers to ignore facts about diet and health in order to further her own agenda: what he calls a controversial, publicity-garnering exposé of the allegedly tobacco-like food industry.

While Milloy sounded fairly convincing, I went ahead anyway and looked up what else Harvard had to say about saturated fats. Here's what I found:

The study Milloy refers to is the Nurses' Health Study; a longitudinal study of diet and lifestyle factors in relation to chronic disease among over 120,000 female registered nurses aged thirty to fifty-five years.

In the November 1997 *New England Journal of Medicine* the same week, Frank Hu, M.D., Ph.D., lead author on the study and research fellow at the Harvard School of Public Health, reported on the results of a large prospective study of nurses, which included over nine hundred cases of heart disease.

The researchers enhanced their ability to examine the associations between fat and the risk of heart disease by taking repeated fat-intake measurements. They found no direct association between total fat intake and the incidence of coronary heart disease. Scientists theorized that this result probably reflected the counterbalancing of different types of fat. When they looked at different types of fats, the picture changed dramatically.

Dr. Hu, the lead author of the study, states, "Our results suggest that replacing saturated and trans fats in the diet with poly and monunsaturated sources of fat is an effective way to reduce coronary heart risk. Reducing overall fat intake is unlikely to affect heart disease risk." The study also found that trans fats are associated with the highest relative risk of coronary heart disease, twice that associated with the same intake of energy from carbohydrates.

It seems that Mr. Milloy may have made a quite liberal interpretation of the study. The study clearly indicates a connection between saturated fats and the "highest relative risk" of coronary heart disease. I don't know how the study he cites could be more clear on the matter.

More recently, Harvard School of Public Health publicized this advice about achieving and maintaining optimal blood cholesterol levels: "You can lower your blood cholesterol level and your risk of heart disease by exercising regularly; maintaining a healthy body weight; increasing dietary fiber; and minimizing the amount of trans fats, limiting the amount of saturated, and replacing these with unsaturated fat and dietary fiber." Again, exactly where is Mr. Milloy getting this idea that Harvard thinks saturated fat is okay? I'm confused.

The saturated fat/heart disease connection isn't the only complaint Milloy has with Dr. Nestle. He also accuses Nestle of having her own concealed bias when it comes to nonprofit groups that frequently comment on food and health issues. He cites the example of the American Council on Science and Health (ACSH). In her book, Nestle derides the ACSH for not disclosing the great extent to which it is funded by food companies. However, Milloy accuses Nestle of hypocrisy for failing to disclose her connections with a rival nonprofit group: the Center for Science in the Public Interest (CSPI). However, he conveniently ignores the important fact that the CSPI is not funded by food companies.

As far as I'm concerned, food companies take issue with the CSPI because it is an honest organization. The CSPI is best known for labeling a dish of fettucine alfredo as a "heart attack on a plate." Of course, such a statement does not go over well with food companies and their supporters, Milloy among them.

What's in a Name?

I'm glad Milloy brought up the CSPI. They are just one of many watchdog trade associations and lobby groups focusing on the food industry.

There's not an issue or commodity that doesn't have a lobby group behind it. Washington, D.C. is chock-full of these groups. Walk the halls of the nation's capital, or any state capital for that matter, and you'll see well-heeled glad-handers clutching glossy brochures and thick wallets. Many of them make their pitch with official sounding names and nutritional studies skewed—naturally—in their favor.

It's not always clear who or what lobby organizations represent. While some food organizations have their product name up front, (such as the sweet, white granular one) others like to portray (disguise) themselves as something other than what they really are. Consider these three organizations frequently cited in articles about specific foods and nutrition:

- International Food Information Council (IFIC)
- Center for Consumer Freedom (CCF)
- American Council on Science and Health (ACSH)

Now, I've got a little quiz for you. See if you can make out the most important differences between these organizations.

Question 1: From its name you can tell this about IFIC:

A. It is dedicated to providing all relevant information about food.
B. If a particular food is bad it will say so.
C. With a name like that, it must be telling the whole, unvarnished story.
D. With a name like that, it would never show bias towards a product.
E. IFIC is supported primarily by the broad-based food, beverage and agricultural industries.

Question 2: From its name you can tell this about CCF:

A. It is dedicated to providing all relevant information about food.
B. If a particular food is bad it will say so.
C. With a name like that, it must be telling the whole, unvarnished story.
D. It is looking out for my right to free choice, and will never show bias towards a product.
E. The CCF is a coalition supported by restaurant operators, food and beverage companies and concerned individuals.

Question 3: From its name you can tell this about ACSH:

A. It is dedicated to providing all relevant information about food.
B. If a particular food is bad it will say so.
C. With a name like that, it must be telling the whole, unvarnished story.
D. It is looking out for my right to free choice, and will never show bias towards a product.
E. ACSH receives financial support from about three hundred different sources, including foundations, trade associations, corporations and individuals.

If you answered "E" to all three questions you'd be right. As for the choices A through D for all three organization, well, those points are open to debate.

Okay, so that was fun. Now let's take a much closer look at each organization. Hopefully this section will help you understand why these groups do what they do.

IFIC

The IFIC (International Food Information Council), which receives its financial support from the food, beverage and agricultural industries, says the mission of its foundation is to convey science-based information on food safety and nutrition to consumers, health professionals, educators, journalists and government officials.

"These groups find the IFIC reservoir of science and health data a valuable and easily accessed resource," it boasts on its Web site.

While the IFIC says its goal is to bridge the informational gap by collecting and disseminating scientific information, what the IFIC fails to reveal are the names of the companies that finance it. It's an impressive list and includes Coca-Cola, Pepsi, Hershey, M&M/MARS Candy and Proctor & Gamble. What conclusions do you think they'd support? Studies disparaging what they sell?

Let's take a look at one example from their literature: caffeine products. If you follow health news regularly, you frequently find research studies about the effects of caffeine. When the news shows a positive—or at least not awful—effect from caffeine, it always has a big caveat: moderate consumption, which frankly represents very little caffeine. Still, when the IFIC publicizes the research it buries or de-emphasizes the "moderation" caveat. When the news is bad, if the IFIC can't spin it, it ignores reporting it entirely.

Here's an example of the IFIC spin from their Web site. In an August 2002 article entitled "Caffeine & Women's Health," the IFIC says even though food products containing caffeine have been enjoyed for a long time, there are those who "question it's safety. But according to leading medical and scientific experts, caffeine in moderation usually can be safely consumed by healthy individuals."

Not to be too critical, the IFIC deserves at least a little credit here. They do use the word *moderation* near the top of the story, but at this point they don't define what moderation means. Is it three cups of coffee? Six cups? Face it; don't we all like to think we use moderation in our behavior—even if it means drinking six to eight cups of coffee in a day?

The IFIC then sets up the premise of the article. "From reproduction to osteoporosis, scientists worldwide have investigated the effects of caffeine on women's health." Finally, a few paragraphs below, they note that moderate caffeine consumption is considered to be about 300 mg., which is equal to around 3 cups of coffee.

Again, here's the rub: the use of the term moderation. The "cup" standard the IFIC uses equals about six to seven ounces of brewed coffee, with each "cup" containing up to 150 mg of caffeine. But who drinks from a six or seven ounce cup? Most people drink from a mug which can easily hold 12 ounces of coffee. That means after one mug you've reached your caffeine quota for the day. That also means you must forego any soft drinks or chocolate—even some medicines containing caffeine. Beyond that, well . . .

They go on: "Overall, individuals tend to find their own acceptable level of caffeine. Those who feel unwanted effects, such as insomnia and the jitters, tend to ease off their caffeine consumption." They make it sound simple and easy. It's not. If you've ever had a caffeine dependency you know there can be withdrawal problems, including torturous headaches.

And buried still further is the key item I believe should be at the very top of the article—if in fact, they want to present critical information about women's health.

"While some studies have shown conflicting results, health professional organizations such as the American College of Obstetricians and Gynecologists recommend that pregnant women limit consumption to the caffeine equivalent of one to two cups of coffee. Use of caffeine in pregnancy should be discussed with health care providers."

Also in the article, the IFIC says it will "provide background information on caffeine and review the latest research on caffeine and women's health, summarizing the major findings . . ."

Well, frankly, they don't. There are many studies the IFIC doesn't mention at all. Here are three recent examples:

Example 1: From Reuters Health, October 25, 2001
"An appetite for coffee and chocolate can take its toll on the bones of elderly women, especially those with a particular genetic mutation, researchers report." Reuters says the elderly women they studied who drank the most coffee had much lower bone mineral density (BMD) after three years compared with women who drank less.

Example 2: From Reuters Health on May 21, 2002
In this article, Reuters reports that two studies unveiled at the American Society of Hypertension's annual meeting showed even small doses of caffeine—as little as the amount found in one to three cups of coffee—can cause temporary stiffening of the blood vessel walls. In one of the studies, from Greece, the researchers found subjects with mild hypertension who took a pill that contained 250 mg of caffeine (an amount equal to 2 to 3 cups of coffee) "experienced a temporary increase in blood pressure and in the stiffness of the aorta, the main artery leaving the heart."

Example 3: From Reuters Health on July 30, 2002

In a study from Duke University in Durham, North Carolina, researchers found that people who consume caffeine experienced an increase in blood pressure, felt more stress and produced more stress hormones than on days when they opt for decaf. Given the long-lasting effects of caffeine, the authors said, "regular consumption of the substance could contribute to the risk of developing heart disease."

Based on these examples, do you think the IFIC's biggest concern is with the caffeine-consuming public or with its clients?

It's not just caffeine the IFIC defends without reservation. Its approach to other foods is the same, but I think you get the picture. In its "Caffeine & Women's Health" study, the IFIC noted it was cosponsored by the Association of Women's Health, Obstetric, and Neonatal Nurses. The IFIC always points out partnerships it says it has forged with a wide range of professional organizations and academic institutions "to develop and disseminate science-based information for the public."

While this seems to add credibility to the research they report, it's important to remember a couple of things. Most important is the "moderation" caveat. No one could argue with the results, unless the moderation part is not emphasized. In this case, I'm sure the Association of Women's Health, Obstetric, and Neonatal Nurses do agree with the results, but the limit on caffeine is the key element, not the inconsequential detail the IFIC chose to present.

A second issue, and frankly I hope I don't sound too cynical here, is many studies are funded by organizations having a vested interest in the results. Face it, some (not all) people or organizations receiving research funding are aware of who is paying for their grant. Unfortunately, we consumers aren't always told who's paying big bucks for scientific studies either.

CCF

On its Web site (www.CCF.org), the Center For Consumer Freedom (CCF) states its membership is comprised of a group of restaurant operators, food and beverage companies—and concerned individuals—"working together to promote personal responsibility and protect consumer choices."

Sounds fair enough, but while the IFIC claims it is disseminating scientific information in the public interest, the CCF's tact approach is very different. They say they're looking out for us, and their tactics are much more in your face.

The CCF says, "Unlike the anti-consumer activists we monitor and keep in check, we stand up for common sense and personal choice. The growing fraternity of 'food cops,' health care enforcers, militant activists, meddling bureaucrats, and violent radicals who think they can decide better than you 'what's best for you' are not just attacking restaurants—they're attacking liberty."

This is how they define consumer freedom; "Consumer freedom is the right of adults and parents to make your own choices about what to do with your money—about what to eat, what to drink, and how to enjoy yourself. We are firm believers in the right to have a good time. Defending enjoyment is what we're all about!"

They continue; "So do we have a bias? You bet we do! We believe that only you know 'what's best for you'—and when activists try to force you to live according to their rules, we don't take it lying down."

The CCF wants to be perceived as tough and brave, speaking up when any "activists proposes curtailing consumer freedom." They say what makes them different from other organizations is "we aren't afraid to take on groups that have built 'good' images through slick public relations campaigns. Remember—even an ugly baby can be named 'Tiffany.' Just because they claim to be 'ethical' or 'responsible' or 'in the public interest' doesn't mean they are."

They also try to portray other adversarial organizations as the evil types who throw bricks through the windows of restaurants and unfairly toss consumers in jail for only having only a couple of alcoholic drinks before driving. The CCF's strategy is to emphasize words and expressions near and dear to our hearts: freedom, personal choice, against restrictions, the rights of parents and adults to choose.

Let's see how they apply that to a controversial subject in a January 2002 article entitled, "Soda and snack foods in schools."

First, they paint California Governor Gray Davis—after he signed into law California Senate Bill 19 on October 13—as focused more on the 2004 presidential election rather than on terrorism and the economy, by fighting such a trivial issue as soda and snack food in schools. The new law, the CCF says, bans the sale of foods "that do not meet arbitrary standards for fat and sugar content on elementary campuses" and limits the sale of carbonated drinks at middle schools. "So, Golden State students, say goodbye to soda with lunch, and to desserts that are more than 35 percent sugar—no matter how healthy a meal they're topping off."

Pointing to how similar freedom-encroaching efforts in other states, besides California, could run rampant through the country brainwashing students with "baseless anti-soda propaganda that links soda consumption to osteoporosis, obesity, tooth decay, and heart disease," the CCF sees this as more an issue of freedom than of health—or soft drink and snack food profits.

"In this latest effort to micromanage schools and students, California's government has actually made things worse. On average, most students buy just two dozen cans of soda from the machines in a school year—less than one can a week . . ."

The CCF points out that schools use the income from soda machines to help pay for extracurricular activities, "those essential parts of the learning experience that are often first on the block during budget-cutting time. In addition, by severely limiting access to soda machines, the law may be stealing some students' best means of getting regular exercise, since soda revenues help pay for athletic programs that taxpayers reject."

The article finishes with this: "Yet (California officials) feel comfortable forcing families and students to accept a Brave New California where classmates bring in boxes of rice cakes to share on their birthdays, douse the coach with a jug of soy milk after winning the homecoming game, and celebrate the end of exams with a big tofu party. Not exactly your memories of youth? With this new law on the books, this could be how today's California children will remember theirs."

I think you get the picture.

ACSH

Here's a summary of American Council on Science and Health (ACSH) standards from its own Web site:

The American Council on Science and Health, Inc. or ACSH

(www.acsh.org), says it is a consumer education consortium concerned with issues related to food, nutrition, chemicals, pharmaceuticals, lifestyle, the environment and health. They claim their independent, nonprofit, tax-exempt organization has a board of 350 physicians, scientists and policy advisors from a wide variety of fields. This board reviews the Council's reports and participate in ACSH seminars, press conferences, media communications and other educational activities

They claim, "Unlike some so-called consumer-advocacy organizations that misrepresent science and distort health priorities, ACSH has a well-established policy of presenting balanced, scientifically sound analyses of current health topics.

"ACSH's is a unique voice, backed by mainstream science, defending the achievements and benefits of responsible technology within America's free-enterprise system."

Right away, you can see some familiar buzz words to prove they're no fringe group: mainstream, defending, responsible, America's free-enterprise system. When I see these words, my guard goes up, (and I hope yours does too).

It ends with a quote which I believe summarizes their whole reason for being. Edwin Feulner, president of the Heritage Foundation, a conservatice think tank, said "On one issue after another in recent years, ACSH has stood as a bulwark against the contemporary Luddites who see the beginning of civilization's end in every technological advance that reaches the market place."

Let's look at one of ACSH's recent positions—this should sound familiar: In a October 1998 article, entitled "Do Sodas Imperil Children's Health?," ACSH said it rejected the Center for Science in the Public Interest's (CSPI) claims that soda necessarily contributes to poor dietary status and/or ill health in children. The fault, they say, lies not with sugary and empty calorie drinks, but with parents that don't take their role or educating their children about proper nutrition. They say there are no good or bad foods, but "dietary immoderation, imbalance and lack of variety."

They point out that consuming too much of anything—even apple juice—is bad for nutrition, since it "crowds out" necessary nutrients from other sources.

Excuse me if I seem impertinent—or unpatriotic—but I have one gargantuan problem with this argument. Anything we consume that contains empty calories replaces something that does. While drinking apple juice might mean we drink less skim milk, drinking soft drinks, which has absolutely no nutritional benefit whatsoever, means we are not gaining the calcium from milk as well as the vitamins from the juice. So which drink is doing the most damage by "crowding out" others? Pul-eeze!

But their arguments don't end with mere variety. "It is counter-productive for a group like CSPI to take on the role of 'food police' and single out specific foods as "bad", says ACSH. "Further it is unreasonable and unjustified for CSPI to target soda manufacturers as the 'villains' when they are A) manufacturing a safe product; and B) it is the role of parents, not corporations, to teach common-sense nutrition habits." To me, it's a modern, skewed version of "let them eat cake."

I can see where someone could ask, "What's the harm in having vending machines at schools dispensing soft drinks? Kids need a little refreshment, and besides, it raises money." As Eric Schlosser points out in his book, *Fast Food Nation*, schools aren't getting that much money from these machines; that is, unless you believe the $27 per student gained by a school in Kansas City is worth inundating children with marketing messages while they slurp syrupy and caffeine-laced products (instead of apple juice!).

Soft drinks aren't as innocent as many believe they are. The National Institute of Diabetes and Digestive and Kidney Diseases (NIDDK) includes cola beverages on a list of foods that doctors may advise patients to avoid especially since they can increase the recurrence of kidney stones. Also, caffeine, a mildly addictive stimulant drug, is added to most colas, Dr. Pepper, some orange sodas, and other soft drinks. Caffeine's addictiveness could be a big reason why six of the seven most popular soft drinks contain caffeine.

Whether it's the dependency on sweetness and/or the caffeine—combined with effective marketing—the soft drink manufacturers are achieving great success. In 1997, Coca-Cola spent $277 million on advertising, and the four major soft-drink companies spent $631 million. Between 1986 and 1997 those companies spent $6.8 billion on advertising. This is the result; according to a study by the "hated" CSPI, in 1978, the average teenage boy drank about seven ounces of soda daily; today he downs three times that amount while deriving nine percent of his daily calories from soft drinks. (During the same period, girls' consumption of soft drinks has doubled.)

Also, while twenty years ago, boys drank twice as much milk as soda, that ratio has now flip-flopped.

Michael S. Finke, an assistant professor or consumer and family economics at the University of Missouri, says the consequences of getting ever more calories from soft drinks or fruit-flavored sugared drinks with no nutrients could be a dangerous trend. Dr. Finke is the author of a study, appearing in the December 2002 issue of the *Family and Consumer Sciences Research Journal* showing more nutrient-rich foods are being replaced by sugar drinks. (One 12-ounce can of cola supplies about 150 calories from about 10 teaspoons of sugar.)

"People haven't really highlighted the consequences of this major food consumption trend," said Dr. Finke. He thinks part of the problem could be simple economics. "Soda pop has always been around, but it's so much cheaper now, relatively speaking, than it was thirty years ago that it is an enticing food option for resource-constrained families." The only cheaper food source, he said, is vegetable oils.

In the study, Finke reviewed the results of a 1994–1996 survey of the USDA's Food Intakes by Individuals, to see if there were any associations between soda consumption and vitamin and mineral deficiency among participants in the self-reported food survey. The scientists looked at fourteen vitamins and minerals. The study did not include information about any vitamin or mineral supplements taken.

"The results were a little bit more dramatic that I had expected," said Dr. Finke. "I expected the results would be significant for nutrients associated with foods that might be replaced by soda, like calcium in milk, but the results were also significant for every other vitamin and mineral."

Finke found that sugar drink consumption was the most consistent variable—more than gender, race, or income—to signal the probability that people would not meet their RDA requirements. The problem, he believes, is not failure to meet RDA requirements, since only a small proportion of the participants actually failed to do so, ranging from 181 people (1.2 percent) for niacin to 1,168 people (7.8 percent) for vitamin A. However, he believes the trend of increased soda pop consumption could increase the likelihood that more people would fail to meet their RDA requirements down the road.

"If someone drinks two cans of soda daily," said Dr. Finke, "which is about 15 percent of daily caloric intake, there is a 1 percent decrease in the probability that the person will meet their RDA requirements in calcium, for instance. So if the trend continues in the future as it has in the past, sugar drink consumption will have an even greater impact on failure to meet RDAs."

Connie Diekman, a nutritionist at the Washington University in St. Louis, agrees that soft drink consumption is a trend threatening to compromise good, nutritional health, especially in young people. "What this study and others have shown is that adolescents increasingly turn to soft drinks for hydration and then don't need to get those calories from healthier choices," she says. "In addition, the long-term effects of inadequate calcium—maybe not deficient, but less than that needed for bone health—are a major health issue."

While ACSH is absolutely, 100 percent correct when they say we should all be free to choose what we put in our bodies, it's important for us to know one thing over and above the impressive lineup of scientists they list on their site. And that is even though they don't mention it—I'm going to guess they forgot—that according to *Consumer Reports*, 40 percent of their funding comes from food industry sources. I think if they were really pressed, they might admit they have a preference for the foods and products that we choose.

CSPI

In case you're keeping score, just as CCF doesn't like CSPI (as illustrated in Steven Milloy's complaint against Nestle's book) there's no love lost for them by ACSH, either. So who is this "disreputable" group, the CSPI?

CSPI, the Center for Science in the Public Interest, is a nonprofit education and advocacy organization (www.cspinet.org). Its goal, it says, is to improve the safety and nutritional quality of our food supply and on "reducing the carnage caused by alcoholic beverages." I'll bet alcohol companies just love this bunch.

At first glance, the goals of CSPI seem in line with the other groups (except about alcohol). It seeks to promote health through educating the public about nutrition and alcohol while representing citizens' interests before legislative, regulatory, and judicial bodies while working to ensure advances in science are used for the public good.

CSPI accepts no corporate or government grants. Instead, it receives its funding from eight hundred thousand subscriptions to its *Nutrition Action Healthletter*—which accepts no advertising—and individual donors. Private foundation grants make up approximately 5 percent to 10 percent of CSPI's annual revenue of $15 million.

In the article, entitled "Liquid Candy," the CSPI gave its own take on soft drinks. It noted in 1997, the soft-drink industry produced fourteen billion gallons of soft drinks, twice as much as in 1974. That equals 576 twelve-ounce servings per year or 1.6 twelve-ounce cans per day for every man, woman and child. To spur sales, the industry increased and heavily marketed the size of servings. In the 1950s, Coca-Cola sold only six-ounce bottles. That was supplanted by twelve-ounce cans. Today, twenty-ounce bottles are becoming the norm.

This means soda has become the average Americans' single biggest source of refined sugars, providing one-third of all sugar. "Because some people drink little soda pop, the percentages are higher among actual drinkers."

CSPI presents other alarming data: most people know it's crucial for females in their teens and twenties to build up bone mass to reduce the risk of osteoporosis later in life. However, according to CSPI, teenage girls consume only 60 percent of the recommended amount of calcium, with soda-pop drinkers consuming almost one-fifth less calcium than nondrinkers. To make matters worse, CSPI says preliminary research suggests that drinking soda pop instead of milk can contribute to broken bones in children and adolescents.

It also notes obesity rates have risen in tandem with soda consumption. Soft drinks provide 10.3 percent of the calories consumed by overweight teenage boys, but only 7.6 percent of the calories consumed by other boys. The National Institutes of Health recommends that people trying to lose or control their weight should drink water instead of soft drinks with sugar.

Quite a difference from the other organizations, wouldn't you say? No wonder so many of us are confused. And these are only a handful of the scores of health-oriented lobby and watchdog groups tying to influence our nutritional policy.

To be fair, all three organizations, IFIC, CCS and ACSH do offer an alternative viewpoint, publicize very good research, have some support from reputable doctors and health associations. But, mixed in are questionable positions and studies reflecting the wishes of their paying clientele more than consumer advocacy. It becomes the difficult task for the consumer to figure out who is serving their best interest.

Regarding the controversy over soft drinks; as you probably realize, the key ingredient is that sweet white stuff I've mentioned before. You know, one of the powerful lobby groups that made life miserable for Marion Nestle.

What's Really Happening

Well, while it's nice to trumpet freedom of choice and the great American desire to keep the government's collective nose out of our business, there's one more thing going on here.

Let me ask you one more question. Do you think it's fair to tell the government to keep its nose out of private affairs, while knocking on a different government door asking for help? Consider this:

> Through its sugar program, the U.S. government guarantees a minimum price to domestic sugar growers by restricting imports and by buying and storing excess production. The result of this intervention is a domestic sugar price that is typically two or three times the world market price. The losers are millions of American families that consume sugar, along with sugar-using industries such as candy-makers, and sugar growers in mostly poor countries.
>
> Also paying the price for the sugar program are taxpayers and the environment. To mop up overproduction caused by price supports and protection, the federal government bought nearly one million tons of sugar last year only to store it in government warehouses. The buying and storing of excess sugar will cost taxpayers an estimated $2 billion over the next ten years. Taxpayers are also paying billions of dollars to help clean up the Florida Everglades, where excess sugar production in the region has disrupted water flows and dumped pollutants such as phosphorus in waterways.

Who wrote this, you ask? It's an article entitled, "Sugar Program Brings Bitter Taste to Holiday Season," written by Daniel T. Griswold, of the Cato Institute. Sound familiar? Ironically, this is the same think tank that employs Mr. Milloy.

Who Funds the CSPI?

Fiscal Year 2002 (July 2001–June 2002)

Allen Foundation, Inc.
Barkley Fund of the Philanthropic Ventures Foundation
Beldon Fund
CECHE (Center for Communications, Health and the
   Environment)
Christopher D. Smithers Foundation, Inc.
Gegax Family Foundation
The Grodzins Fund
Helena Rubinstein Foundation
Homeland Foundation
The Irving & Edyth S. Usen Family Charitable
   Foundation
The Joyce Foundation
The John Merck Fund
New York Community Trust
Park Foundation, Inc.
Myra Reinhard Family Foundation
The Robert Wood Johnson Foundation
Rockefeller Family Fund, Inc.
The Rockefeller Foundation
Saperstein Family Fund
Szekely Family Foundation
Wallace Genetic Foundation

As I hope you can see, setting nutritional standards aren't all that easy. There are a lot of factors—and players—at work. (And we haven't even gotten to the infamous Food Pyramid yet—perhaps the greatest source of nutrition confusion.)

If you're still unsure—or confused—about the value of our nutritional standards and whether they're working, I'll repeat what I suggested earlier. The next time you're in a public place, look to your left and look to your right. You should have your answer.

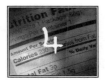

Pyramid Schemes

Think about it. There is probably no industry more important to Americans, more fundamentally linked to our health, than the food industry. And, the nutritional standard with the greatest influence on us—above and beyond the RDAs or DRIs and the official Dietary Guidelines—is probably the infamous USDA Food Guide Pyramid.

Food Guide Pyramid designers thought that by featuring common foods, more people would use the pyramid to actually achieve a balanced diet. But some researchers are not happy with the nutritional message of the USDA pyramid. They think that the government's recommendations rely too heavily on animal foods, refined grains, and give "heart healthy" vegetables, fruits, and other whole foods too little recognition.

To recap, the Dietary Guidelines for Americans were developed to set good dietary practices for individuals and families. The Dietary Guidelines for Americans is a publication issued jointly by two agencies of the U.S. government, the United States Departments of Health and Human Services (HHS) and Agriculture (USDA). This document provides a variety of tools to assist with diet planning.

According to the HHS and USDA, "It [the Food Guide Pyramid] is the product of a thorough process of collecting scientific research about diet and nutrition and then using the research findings to help develop federal nutrition policy. Based on this information, the Guidelines offer adults and children over two years of age sound advice about how good dietary habits may reduce the chance of acquiring chronic diseases or illnesses."

In addition to the pyramid and the Dietary Guidelines for Americans, the DRIs the RDAs, and the three other nutrient indicators—the Estimated Average Requirement, the Tolerable Intake Level and the Adequate Intake—round out the tools the HHS and the USDA provide to assist with diet planning.

Back to the Pyramid

The original four food groups have been a familiar nutritional staple for decades. The Food Guide Pyramid, which expanded the number of food groups to five then six, was developed by the USDA in 1992.

While items in the pyramid have been shuffled around from time to time, the current Food Guide Pyramid recommends the following six categories of foods:

- 6 to 11 servings of bread, cereal, rice and pasta
- 3 to 5 servings of vegetables
- 2 to 4 servings of fruits
- 2 to 3 servings of milk, yogurt and cheese
- 2 to 3 servings of meat, poultry, fish, dry beans, eggs and nuts
- Fats, oils and sweets used sparingly

Today the guidelines, including the Food Guide Pyramid, are prominent features on food labels, in elementary school cafeterias, on walls in doctors' offices and in certain fast food restaurants, and are also referenced by physicians, nutritionists and even grocery shoppers.

These guidelines determine all federal food-assistance programs, including the National School Lunch and Breakfast Programs, the Food Stamp Program, and the Women, Infants, and Children Supplemental Feeding Program (WIC).

The Food Guide Pyramid establishes some basic rules, such as the recommended number of servings of each food, and guides individuals about the amount of fats and sugars that are likely to be in a certain types of food.

Sounds good, right? Then why are we getting fatter and—as many health experts and organizations say—more prone to many illnesses?

What if, let's say beginning today, we all started to follow the U.S. Dietary Guidelines, including the well-known Food Guide Pyramid? Would we see slimmer people and dramatic decreases in chronic diseases? Not likely.

Rather than being the standard for sound nutrition, many industry observers say the Food Guide Pyramid is an example of how the food industry pressures government nutrition policies and how cleverly it links its interests to those of nutrition experts. Walter C. Willett, M.D., author of the *Harvard Medical School Guide to Healthy Eating*, says by promoting the USDA Food Pyramid, the Department of Agriculture—the agency with the dual responsibilities of promoting the products of American agribusiness, while also monitoring and protecting our health—is serving two often conflicting masters. While it's supposed to sort out and inform us of the latest sound nutritional information, it tries to do so while listening to the persuasive and well-connected representatives of powerful lobby groups such as the meat, dairy and sugar industries.

The end result, says Willett, are recommendations that distort and compromise possibly the most important nutritional guidelines we have. At best, says Willett, the USDA pyramid offers indecisive, scientifically unfounded advice on an absolutely vital topic— what to eat. At worst, the misinformation it offers contributes to weight gain, poor health, and unnecessary early deaths.

But it's not just lobby groups that influence the government. Many of the "experts" who created these guidelines have historically been financial partners with the meat, dairy and egg producers.

Nearly a Century's Worth of Advice

Let's back up. As I've said, the first USDA food guide was published in 1916 with several other guides published during the next thirty years.

In the early 1950s, the USDA created four food groups:

- milk
- meat
- fruits and vegetables
- breads and cereals

Called the "Basic Four," this list was the first time the U.S. government specified the number and size of suggested food servings. Since they had a vested interest in the guidelines, it's no surprise food industry representatives played an integral part in devising this new plan. In fact, the National Dairy Council was so pleased with the guidelines that it distributed its own version as a public service.

The Basic Four remained virtually unchanged for the next thirty-five years. Then in the 1970s, as a result of new disease and nutrition studies, scientists made new dietary recommendations to reduce the risks of heart disease and other diet-related illnesses. The suggested changes included much lower intake levels of overall fat and especially cholesterol, which is found only in animal products. Needless to say, some food industries stewed over the proposed changes.

In 1977, the Senate Select Committee on Nutrition and Human Needs published *Dietary Goals for the United States*, a report advising the reduction of cholesterol, saturated fat, and total fat, along with consumption of more fruits, vegetables, and whole grains. Under pressure from cattlemen and dairy farmers, the report was revised a few months later to change its message from "eat less meat and milk" to "choose lean meat and nonfat milk."

Then, in 1980, the USDA published the first official Dietary Guidelines for Americans, based largely on the Dietary Goals report. As soon as the new guidelines were released, the meat and dairy industries objected—fearful that as the public became aware of new information regarding fat and cholesterol, consumption of animal products would be threatened. An advisory committee was appointed to make revisions. Agricultural producers responded by increasing political lobbying in an attempt to discredit the new federal dietary recommendations.

Despite political pressure, by the early 1980s, USDA officials began working on a new model to replace the Basic Four: one that would ensure adequate intake of fiber, which is found only in plants, and recommend less fat and cholesterol than the previous plan.

In 1989, the USDA came up with the "Eating Right Pyramid," which emphasized grains and other plant foods at the pyramid's base and which de-emphasized animal products by putting these products at the top.

Sent to thirty-six nutritional experts and presented at numerous professional conferences, the pyramid received widespread approval. However, several weeks before the pyramid was to be released in April 1991, the Physicians Committee for Responsible Medicine (PCRM) asked the USDA to replace the Basic Four with the New Four Food Groups:

- whole grains
- vegetables
- legumes
- fruits

Founded in 1985, the Physicians Committee for Responsible Medicine promotes preventive medicine and higher standards in medical research, education, and practice. PCRM is a nonprofit organization based in Washington, D.C. (See sidebar on next page.)

In response to the New Four, the meat, dairy and egg lobbyists went into battle mode. Within days, and clutching their own medical studies, members of the National Cattlemen's Association met with the new Secretary of Agriculture, Edward R. Madigan, and complained about the upcoming release of the Eating Right Pyramid, claiming that the new pyramid would hurt beef sales. The National Milk Producers Federation and other trade associations joined the Cattlemen's Association in fighting the publication of the new model.

Within weeks, the Eating Right Pyramid was withdrawn with Secretary Madigan saying it was "confusing to children." After conferring with lobbyists and USDA employees, PCRM said the real reason it was withdrawn due to industry pressure. The American Cancer Society, the American Medical Association and other health and medical organizations protested with little success.

But the USDA wasn't done yet. In July 1991, it hired another private firm to determine if the pyramid was better than other designs, such as a bowl. The agency said it wanted the symbol tested on USDA's target audiences of children and those with minimal education. After months of costly analysis and market research, the USDA again settled on the pyramid.

The Physicians Committee for Responsible Medicine (PCRM)

PCRM president Neal D. Barnard, M.D., is the author of *Turn Off the Fat Genes; Foods That Fight Pain; Eat Right, Live Longer; Food for Life;* and other books on preventive medicine.

As of December 2002, PCRM's advisory board includes twelve health care professionals from a broad range of specialties. Many of these names should be familiar to you.

T. Colin Campbell, Ph.D., Cornell University
Caldwell B. Esselstyn, Jr., M.D., The Cleveland Clinic
Suzanne Havala, Ph.D., M.S., R.D., L.D.N., F.A.D.A., The Vegetarian Resource Group
Henry J. Heimlich, M.D., Sc.D., The Heimlich Institute
Lawrence Kushi, Ph.D., University of Minnesota
Virginia Messina, M.P.H., R.D., Nutrition Matters, Inc.
John McDougall, M.D., McDougall Program, St. Helena Hospital
Milton Mills, M.D., Gilead Medical Group
Dean Ornish, M.D., Preventive Medicine Research Institute
Myriam Parham, R.D., L.D., C.D.E., East Pasco Medical Center
William Roberts, M.D., Baylor Cardiovascular Institute
Andrew Weil, M.D., University of Arizona

When the pyramid was released in April 1992—a year later than expected—there were thirty-three changes, many based on demands from the meat and dairy industries.

From 1992 to 1995, food producers continued their active political lobbying, trying to influence the revision of the Dietary Guidelines for Americans. Minor changes were made in 1995.

While leading nutrition experts promoted the idea that the best, and possibly easiest, way to stay slim and lower the risk for many diseases is to eat a diet rich in plant foods, the federal government, clings to other ideas and, some would say, agendas.

Despite scientific evidence that meat- and dairy-heavy diets contribute to serious health problems including obesity, diabetes, stroke, heart disease, and cancer, the government continued to promote four to six daily servings of animal products as necessary for good health. For certain ethnic groups such as African-, Asian-, and Hispanic-Americans, that are largely lactose-intolerant, the result is particularly bad. Long touted as the best calcium source, the fact is, dairy products can wreak digestive havoc on the nation's African-, Asian-, Hispanic- and Native Americans. Studies show as many as 95 percent of Asian Americans, 70 percent of African Americans and Native Americans, and the majority of Hispanic Americans simply cannot digest the sugar in cow's milk. Yet, like every other "average" American, they are told eat dairy products even though their cultures rarely or never consume milk products and have much lower rates of osteoporosis than in the United States.

In 1998, the USDA and the HHS announced the appointment of the fifth Dietary Guidelines Advisory Committee, which was scheduled to recommend further revisions to the guidelines before January 2000, with the fifth edition released in midyear. But there was trouble brewing.

PCRM wasn't ready to quit. While they agreed it's every American's right to shun nutritional guidelines if they wish, if the government insists on formulating dietary guidelines, the PCRM should serve as the superlative model for good nutrition—featuring only those foods that are essential and health promoting.

Before the 2000 guidelines could be released, PCRM did some snooping around, looking at the Dietary Guidelines Advisory Committee, the folks who have the final say on the standards. They were not surprised to discover a high level of influence by the meat, dairy and egg industries. For example, committee chair Cutberto Garza has worked closely with the National Dairy Council, Mead Johnson Nutritionals (a major seller of dairy-based products) and the Nestlé Company, and has served as a scientific adviser to a Dannon yogurt affiliate. At least six of the eleven committee members have major ties to groups such as the National Dairy Promotion and Research Board, the National Live Stock and Meat Board, SlimFast Nutrition Institute, the American Egg Board Grant Review Committee, and the American Meat Institute. All these officals were appointed by the USDA and the U.S. Department of Health and Human Services.

According to Mindy S. Kursban, an attorney for PCRM, it's not only unethical to stack this committee with individuals who have an economic stake in their own recommendations, it's against federal law. "In 1972, Congress strictly prohibited industry influence over government policies via advisory committees," Kursban said. "The law aimed at eliminating special interests, ensuring fair representation of viewpoints, and encouraging public access and participation within such committees. Sadly, USDA itself felt justified in employing Eileen Kennedy as its Deputy Under Secretary of Agriculture while she worked as a scientific adviser with the same Dannon affiliate as Garza."

In December 1999, PCRM filed a lawsuit in U.S. District Court in Washington, D.C. arguing that at least six of the eleven members of the Dietary Guidelines Advisory Committee had financial ties to the meat, dairy, or egg industries. Such ties may have made it more likely that unhealthy foods would remain in the government's diet plan. PCRM's suit also charged that the government had undercut the public's ability to participate in and understand the committee's activities.

Prior to initiating the lawsuit, PCRM's efforts to change federal diet guidelines had won the support of the NAACP, former Surgeon General Joycelyn Elders, Martin Luther King III, Muhammad Ali, and many others who objected to the over-promotion of meat and dairy products given the prevalence of lactose intolerance and diet-related diseases, such as heart disease, diabetes, and hypertension, among racial minorities.

The doctors' group scored a partial victory in February, when the advisory committee accepted nondairy foods, such as soymilk, as acceptable alternatives to dairy products. But that was only the beginning. The following October, U.S. District Judge James Robertson said the USDA violated federal law by keeping secret certain documents used in setting federal nutrition policies and by hiding financial conflicts of interest among members of the diet advisory committee.

While the USDA had provided information showing financial conflicts of interest for six committee members, Judge Robertson faulted the department for refusing to provide details on an additional conflicts of interest, including a payment of more than $10,000 for one member. "Having advisors tied to the meat or dairy industries is as inappropriate as letting tobacco companies decide our standards for air quality," said PCRM president Neal D. Barnard, M.D.

Kursban, PCRM's attorney, said, "We hope that this Court's strong ruling against the government will make the USDA think twice before appointing Committee members with inappropriate industry ties."

Kursban believes the lawsuit will insure that future committee members are selected based on professional expertise and free of bias. She realizes the lawsuit victory was only a first step toward this goal. "All eyes will be on future advisory committees, ensuring that members are free of inappropriate financial motivations. Only then will ALL Americans get a fair shot at receiving sound, unbiased nutritional advice," Kursban said.

It's Not Just Fat

In the early 1900s heart attacks were rare. Today it's practically an epidemic. While "bad" fat and cholesterol play a huge role, there's another substance—with a powerful lobby behind it that has helped sway our government nutritional guidelines. Yeah, that white, sweet granular stuff, which after it is refined has no nutritional value and if consumed in excess, is converted from a carbohydrate to fat and is stored in the body.

What does this have to do with the current food pyramid? Prior to 1991, the obesity rate in this country was 25 percent of the population. Today, 57 percent of Americans are classified as clinically obese. Why? The answer is quite simple. The food pyramid advocates a diet heavily overloaded with carbohydrates.

In the past few decades, modern technology has drastically increased the production of grains in this country. In the early 1990s, as many of us learned about the dangers of fatty meats, we were urged to eat more grains. Low-fat foods flooded the market. Unfortunately, reducing the amount of fat in foods makes them taste terrible. Therefore, low-fat foods are often loaded up with sugar to make them palatable. A simple hot dog, which used to be pure protein and had no carbohydrates, now has an average of 2 grams of carbohydrates. "Low-fat" hotdogs now have as much as 6 grams of carbohydrates each—all from added sugar. The same is true with all products labeled "low fat."

Many of us bought into this new diet and every year we got bigger and more of us died. Studies from Harvard, Stanford and other major universities have proven that this type of diet is deadly, increases heart disease and leads to stroke and diabetes.

Maybe it's just a coincidence, but the new emphasis on carbs was introduced at exactly the same time that the USDA was paying gigantic subsidies to American farmers to plow under their products.

Of course, not all carbs are the same, as you'll see in a later chapter. Suffice it to say the Food Guide Pyramid has had us bulk up on carbs both in the "bread, cereal, rice, & pasta" group, as well as the complex carbohydrate "fruits and vegetable" group, which is the preferred method of fueling up—and the most ignored.

Another Solution for Outside Influences

Even though PCRM won its court case, obviously we haven't seen the Food Guide Pyramid changed as a result. Hopefully, we will see meaningful change in the future.

The controversy over how food research is presented, usually supported by "scientific studies," raises doubts about how authentic some of these studies are. Many in the scientific community have noticed.

I don't think anyone could reasonably disagree that when dealing with issues as important as medical research that will affect people's lives it is of the utmost importance that the data be accurate—and the conclusions drawn from them be completely unbiased. The reality is university-based educators and researchers, as well as private practitioners, are in frequent contact with representatives from for-profit companies that provide "gifts" and financial support for teaching and research.

Writing in the *Journal of the American Medical Association* in 2000, Dr. J.P. Kassirer said enticement begins very early in a physician's career. "For my classmates and me, it started with black bags."

Dr. Kassirer said the timing of presenting the black bags early in the first year was wonderfully strategic, as was the inscription of their names on each. "I must admit I was very happy to finally have a real symbol of the medical profession after so many hours of what seemed like year five of college. On the other hand, at that time I did not have the courage to publicly state my unease with the unearned 'gift.'" While Dr. Kassirer's article referred to gifts from pharmaceutical companies, the same can be said for food lobbyists also.

Subsequently, Dr. Kassirer said offers came for "free" lunches, dinners, and tickets to various events followed by offers to serve as an "expert" with the usual lineup of speaking engagements and serving on advisory panels and boards, for an "honorarium" of course. "There should be little question about the expected effects of accepting free food, tickets and even black bags. It has been shown that clinicians' decisions are affected by their interactions with pharmaceutical companies," says Kassirer.

The problem, he says, lies in conflicts of interest resulting from these relationships. "However, it is vitally important to understand that a conflict of interest does not necessarily result in an outcome different than the result would have been without such conflict."

Still, appearances are everything. A study appearing in *USA Today* on September 25, 2000 showed more than half of the advisors to the Food and Drug Administration (FDA) have financial relationships with pharmaceutical companies that have an interest in FDA decisions.

Dr. Kassirer says when an investigator has a financial interest in or funding by a company with activities related to his or her research, the research is

- lower in quality
- more likely to favor the sponsor's product
- less likely to be published
- more likely to have delayed publication

Dr. Kassirer said those best prepared and experienced to carry out complex studies generally are faculty in academic institutions. Unfortunately, since there is little chance that sufficient funding for important clinical research—especially expensive clinical trials—will be forthcoming from sources other than sponsors with a vested interest in the results, the only hope is for institutional safeguards to be implemented to mitigate the negative effects of funding from companies with a vested interest in the results.

"It is vitally important that these institutions develop conflict-of-interest policies, have oversight mechanisms in place, and continuously monitor the relationships of faculty with sponsoring companies and agencies," said Dr. Kassirer.

"Without these policies and procedures, the academic institutions where most clinical research is based (and their faculty members who perform the research) are in grave danger of losing the support and respect of the public. Without this support and respect, trust in new medical discoveries and their applications will not be forthcoming." He added, " Without trust, medical research is doomed."

Towards a Better Pyramid

There's a new pyramid scheduled to come out in 2003. Hopefully it will be free of political influence and will depend on sound nutritional advice by experts without agendas. Some scientists and nutritional experts are full of suggestions about what it should look like. Some have even made their own pyramids.

For example, Harvard University's Dr. Walter Willet has devised his own pyramid which included the following:

Exercise at the Base

Daily exercise and weight control are the foundations of Willett's pyramid. Since we now know inactivity contributes to many chronic disease such as diabetes, heart disease, obesity and osteoporosis, we all need to focus on getting more exercise—preferably with activities we enjoy.

Good Fats and Whole Grains

Dr. Willet believes next in line for better health are good fats and whole grains. The bread, cereal, rice and pasta group that appears at the base of the original pyramid is high in carbohydrates, the body's primary source of fuel. In addition, grain products are high in fiber, minerals, and other vitamins.

But, he notes, the USDA Pyramid ignores the fact that the most common grain products on grocery store shelves—white bread, crackers, pasta, and cereal—are made with refined flour that has lost nutrients during processing. As a result, one of the biggest shortcomings of the USDA pyramid is that it fails to distinguish between a plateful of pasta and a bowl of whole-grain oats.

Some scientists believe a diet high in refined grain foods like white rice, potatoes, and products made from white flour, may actually be fueling the rapid increase in diabetes, heart disease, and obesity. If that's true, it's not the carbohydrates themselves that are responsible for any ill health effects, but the form that they come in. One theory, put forth by Tufts researcher, Susan B. Roberts, states that refined carbohydrates cause a rapid rise in blood insulin, a hormone that keeps blood sugar levels in control. Many researchers believe that consuming too much of these foods over time taxes our systems and makes us more prone to diabetes and heart disease. Whole-grain foods such as whole wheat, brown rice and oatmeal, on the other hand, are good sources of fiber, which slows the release of carbohydrates into the bloodstream and keeps insulin levels from spiking.

The scientists say keeping insulin on an even keel is key to weight control. Whole grains also contain many phytochemicals that experts believe help to maintain good health.

Willet says unlike the USDA pyramid, which places fat at the top to be consumed in very limited quantities, fat really belongs at the very bottom of the pyramid, right next to whole grains. But not all fats. Since saturated fats from meat and dairy foods can contribute to the development of heart disease, they should be shunned. Vegetable oils such as olive and canola, on the other hand, may well deserve a prominent place in the American diet. These monounsaturated and polyunsaturated fats are considered "heart healthy" because they do not raise blood cholesterol levels and may even help slow the progression of heart disease. This notion of good versus bad fats is supported by the fact that Mediterranean cultures that consume a high amount of plant oils and fatty fish have very little incidence of diabetes and heart disease.

Vitamins, Minerals, Fiber and Phytochemicals

Once our basic energy needs have been met, the group of foods we should focus on comes from vegetables and fruits. Eaten in abundance these foods provide essential vitamins and minerals and enough fiber and disease-fighting phytochemicals to help keep you healthy. Although the standard recommendation is five servings a day, no one will argue that the more you get, the better. In fact, Tufts scientist, Jim Joseph, recommends up to nine servings a day to reduce the risk of cancer and other age-related diseases. To get the most from your servings, choose leafy greens regularly, lots of berries, and shoot for maximum color diversity. Every color of fruit and/or vegetable will deliver unique health benefits.

Nuts and Legumes

Not only do nuts provide high-quality protein, they also come packed with "good" fats; i.e., fats that help lower "bad" cholesterol. And beans are another good source of protein, with the added value of fiber, which helps control appetite, may help reduce the risk of heart disease, and may even fight cancer.

Fish, Poultry, and Eggs

The USDA pyramid puts nuts, legumes, red meat, fish and eggs all in one category, suggesting that they are all equal. But research shows they are indeed very different. Unlike red meat, fish has almost no artery-clogging saturated fat, but it has lots of "essential fats," the kind of fats that help make important hormones that regulate body functions and may help prevent heart attacks. Eggs are also getting another look as a good source of protein—new research shows that an egg a day is not bad for your heart. Furthermore, egg yolks contain phytochemicals—lutein and zeanxanthin—that help fight age-related cataracts.

Dairy

A growing school of thought in the nutrition community says it's not necessary to rely solely on dairy foods for calcium. These experts point to evidence that many Americans' diets lack the minerals needed for calcium balance.

According to research by Katherine Tucker of Tufts University, if we focused more on whole foods, such as whole grains, legumes, and produce, we would create a positive mineral balance and easily meet our daily calcium needs. Not all plant foods contain calcium, though, so have some good alternative sources of calcium, such as soy-based products and calcium-fortified orange juice, before you ditch dairy from your diet.

Willett's revised pyramid lumps red meat, butter, white rice, white bread, potatoes, pasta, and sweets into one category at the very tip of the pyramid, only to be used sparingly. Red meat and butter contain a lot of harmful saturated fat, whereas potatoes, refined grain products and sweets contain "empty calories" that may contribute to weight gain and diabetes.

Not all scientists believe potatoes and pasta are bad for you, but most agree that loading up on one kind of food (like pasta) while shunning other kinds of foods (like vegetables) is an unhealthy way to eat. Regardless of how they package it, though, their nutrition advice is basically the same: eat a diet high in fruits, vegetables, and whole-grain foods, eat less red meat and more fish, choose low-fat dairy foods if you include dairy in your diet, and go with vegetable oils and spreads over animal fats like butter.

One Size Doesn't Fit All

Since a basic premise of this book is that one nutritional size should not fit all, then the food pyramid should be modified for special needs. One obvious case is older people.

Food Pyramid for Elderly People

Many of the ailments afflicting older people can be traced directly or indirectly to poor nutrition. It's no secret, often due to financial considerations, that large numbers of elderly Americans fall seriously short of nutritional recommendations, consuming the least nutritious choices in each food category, like white bread instead of whole grain and fruit juice instead of whole fruit. Also, as energy needs decline with age, the elderly tend to eat fewer calories, and hence fewer servings, of the recommended food groups.

Dr. Robert M. Russell, a professor of medicine and nutrition at Tufts University and his colleagues at the Department of Agriculture's Human Nutrition Research Center on Aging have developed a revised food guide pyramid for Americans over seventy. Their guide was published in the March 1999 issue of the *Journal of Nutrition*.

One key element of their guide is a new foundation: water, eight 8-ounce glasses each day. Dr. Russell explained that without enough water, blood pressure can fall dangerously low, clots may form and block blood vessels, kidney function may be compromised (and may result in toxic concentrations of drugs) and constipation can become chronic. "Older people have a reduced thirst mechanism," Dr. Russell told the *New York Times*. "They have to consciously think of drinking more and keeping well hydrated, especially if they live in warm climates."

Dr. Russell also recommends that on the next level of this elderly pyramid should include six or more servings a day of grain-based foods like bread, cereal, rice and pasta, which form the bulk of the elderly diet—with an emphasis on fiber-rich choices. Fiber helps prevent constipation, diverticulosis and diverticulitis.

Certain fibers also counter high cholesterol, protect against cancer and maintain a normal blood sugar level, which is especially important for people with diabetes. Also, the cereals should be fortified with extra nutrients, especially B vitamins like folic acid and B12. (Folic acid can lower blood levels of homocysteine, a substance that increases the risk of heart disease.)

Next come fruits and vegetables, which are best consumed as fiber-rich whole foods, not juice. They can be sliced, chopped or puréed, and they can be fresh, canned or frozen, but fruits packed in syrup provide too many sweet calories. Also, the recommended three or more servings of vegetables and two or more servings of fruits should include foods that are richly colored—dark green, orange, red or yellow. These are richest in essential nutrients. In addition, vegetables in the cabbage family like broccoli, cauliflower, kale and mustard greens are rich in cancer-blocking chemicals.

Dr. Russell says for the dairy group, the three recommended servings a day should feature low-fat choices. Dr. Russell noted that people who were lactose intolerant could still consume lactose-reduced milk, low-fat hard cheeses and yogurt.

As for the meat group, the two or more daily servings should emphasize variety and feature fish (which may reduce cardiac risk) and dried beans (which are rich in fiber) as well as lean cuts of meat and poultry.

The Tufts researchers say the consumption of high-fat and highly sweetened foods should be limited since they provide nutritionally empty calories and leave less room in the daily energy quotient for nutrient-rich foods. As for the types of fats used in cooking, in dressings and as table spreads, the Tufts scientists recommend liquid oils and, if margarine is used it should be free of the so-called trans fatty acids.

There's something else in the elderly pyramid never seen in the traditional one: supplements. The Tufts researchers treat it as a sort of "flag" at the peak. Dr. Russell explained that few older people are able to get enough calcium, vitamin B12 and vitamin D from their diets to achieve the recommended intake of these nutrients, and many would have to take supplements to fulfill these nutritional needs.

Dr. Russell says based on studies of bone metabolism over the last two decades, older people are now being advised to consume 400 IU of vitamin D daily, which is double the previous recommendation and is equal to the amount found in a quart of milk. Although vitamin D is made in the skin when it is exposed to sunlight, many older people do not spend enough time outdoors to meet their need for this nutrient.

It is also difficult for the elderly to achieve the recommended intake of calcium (1,200 to 1,400 mg a day—up from 800 mg), which is also about the same as found in a quart of milk.

As for vitamin B12, a diet containing any animal foods supplies this nutrient. But among people over sixty, Russell said 10 percent to 30 percent do not form enough acid in their stomachs to release the vitamin from the food protein that binds it. If the vitamin remains bound, it cannot be absorbed. B12 that can be absorbed even by people with low stomach acid is found in supplements and in cereals fortified with the vitamin.

Nutrition and the First Amendment

Here's the latest skirmish we consumers are facing: Do food companies—or any organizations for that matter—have a First Amendment right to promote their products as they see fit?

The First Amendment to the Constitution says: "Congress shall make no law respecting an establishment of religion, or prohibiting the free exercise thereof; or abridging the freedom of speech, or of the press; or the right of the people peaceably to assemble, and to petition the government for a redress of grievances." In this case, we're talking about the "abridging the freedom of speech" part of the amendment along with "and to petition the government for a redress of grievances."

That's the current battle that's raging. Face it, as I've said before we are no match for clever advertising. It's very hard for us to evaluate a product if we don't have all the facts. Although nondisclosure of important information might be a critical part of Marketing 101—emphasizing your product's strengths while avoiding mention of its flaws—might not technically be lying, it is disingenuous.

Here's where we stand in the battle. After losing a series of court decisions that found it in violation of the First Amendment's guarantee of freedom of speech, the Food and Drug Administration has begun a wide-ranging review of regulations that control what the makers of foods, drugs, supplements and cosmetics can say about their products. At issue is the delicate balance between a company's right to communicate with its customers and the food and drug agency's mandate to protect the public.

But the court decisions, which included a stinging rebuke from the Supreme Court in April 2002, have prompted the agency to ask whether it may, at times, have gone too far in its insistence that it decides when scientific truth has been established and what companies can say. Until now, the agency's position has been that it decides what companies can say and how they can say it. Its mission of protecting the public health, the agency argued, gives it broad authority to regulate commercial speech, including misleading product claims.

To explore this issue, the government published a notice in *The Federal Register* on May 16, 2002, inviting interested parties to comment on "First Amendment issues." Hundreds replied, with wish lists, cries of alarm and hefty documents.

Dr. David A. Kessler, who was the agency's commissioner from 1990 to 1997 and is now the dean of Yale's School of Medicine, says the effort by some represents a frontal attack on the fundamental responsibilities of the agency under the Food, Drug and Cosmetic Act. "I have great concerns that this is simply an attempt to deregulate while doing it in the name of the First Amendment," Kessler told the *New York Times* on October 15, 2002.

Dr. Rhona Applebaum, executive vice president for scientific and regulatory affairs at the National Food Processors Association, describes agency regulations as "command and control." "The way it stands now, any type of implied disease benefit, the agency throws it into our faces."

In one instance, said Dr. Applebaum, while studies suggest that dietary calcium is associated with lower blood pressure the FDA does not find the evidence conclusive. Applebaum told the *New York Times*, that food manufacturers would be happy to put in disclaimers, such as "While inconclusive, new research seems to indicate . . ." or "Preliminary evidence suggests that calcium promotes healthy blood pressure. But right now we can't say it."

David Vladeck is a lawyer who heads the litigation group for Public Citizen, a consumer advocacy group which accepts no government or corporate money. He says that there are real questions here, but that does not mean the answer is to deregulate.

Public Citizen notes the official position of the Supreme Court has repeatedly been against misleading commercial speech and that it can be regulated without running afoul of the First Amendment. The Court states, "In the area of food and drug law, health claims unsupported by significant and reputable scientific evidence are unreliable and misleading."

The consumer watchdog group also notes that wherever public health is threatened by such claims, they can be suppressed in their entirety. Public Citizen says, "Government can serve no more important role than to level the information playing field. This is a function that has not been effectively filled by the FDA, and the FDA's ability to do so has now been called into question by this request for comment."

In this instance we have a clash between a slow and cautions government agency under extreme pressure from many fronts and the interest of companies wanting maximum leverage to sell their products.

For true consumer clarity might we need to look beyond the fact that the product seldom looks—or tastes—as advertised and accept that cleverly concocted product names like *down home, hearth, country*, and *nature* are simply gimmicks.

I'll repeat the facts I stated earlier: "The food industry actively promotes overeating by spending $10 billion a year in direct media advertising. It also spends another $20 billion a year in indirect marketing, including things like toy prizes, sponsorships or sporting events logos on school scoreboards."

Let's look at the way the food industry has marketed the fat substitute Olestra. When first announced, everyone was excited about it because of the possibility it would help people eat diets lower in fat (especially saturated fat) and prevent obesity and heart disease. But there were some problems.

Here are a few of the problems the Center for Science in the Public Interest noted soon after Olestra was introduced: Olestra rapidly depletes blood levels of many valuable fat-soluble substances, including carotenoids. Supplementing olestra with selected vitamins will not solve all of olestra's nutrient-depletion problems. "Olestra is highly effective at reducing serum levels of the fat-soluble vitamins A, D, E, and K," states a CSPI report. "Simply supplementing olestra with those vitamins, as Procter & Gamble has proposed, would not completely solve that problem."

Olestra causes gastrointestinal disturbances, which are sometimes severe, including diarrhea, fecal urgency, and more frequent and looser bowel movements. CSPI reports that a variety of gastrointestinal symptoms occurred in subjects who consumed on a daily basis the amount of Olestra that would be found in less than one ounce of potato chips (about sixteen chips), as well as higher doses. Olestra sometimes causes underwear staining associated with "anal leakage." Want a fat-free potato chip?

Data is lacking on the health effects of Olestra on potentially vulnerable segments of the population. Key tests were unacceptably brief. "Only poor studies have examined the effect of Olestra on gastrointestinal disturbances in children, while no studies at all have focused on gastrointestinal problems and nutrient losses in healthy people over forty-four years of age and people with poor nutritional status."

Procter & Gamble's claim that Olestra's gastrointestinal effects are similar to those caused by high-fiber diets is not true.

Of course this is just one side of the story. But isn't this information important enough for us to have so we, on our own, can weigh the risks versus the benefits? Deciding whether or not we're willing to exercise our freedom of choice requires us to have all the facts.

If, as the American Council on Science and Health claims, "ACSH has stood as a bulwark against the contemporary Luddites who see the beginning of civilization's end in every technological advance that reaches the market place," meaning CSPI critique of products such as Olestra is the result of its own agenda, don't we need to know this also?

Hopefully, and ideally, when we strip away all the legalese, the First Amendment issue will be decided by the underlying principals of honesty and integrity and the First Amendment rights of corporations aren't greater than the individual. Hopefully our health won't be compromised by what is in the best interest of lobby groups, trade associations or bureaucrats. And in an ideal world, half-truths or the purposeful omitting of facts is just as wrong as flat-out lying.

True Freedom of Choice

Instead, what "we the people" need and deserve, is the most accurate, up-to-date and unvarnished information. We must all weigh, individually and collectively, our comfort levels of "free choice" and "consumer protection." After all, it's our country and our FDA.

Obviously there are flaws in our government's methods of implementing standards. But if the government doesn't do it, who should? One side says industry should be allowed to self-regulate itself. In an October 2002 editorial in the *Atlanta Journal and Constitution*, Yaron Brook, executive director of the Ayn Rand Institute, argues that America's businessmen are the "productive dynamos that move our economy forward." Brooks says "they have brought us from horse and buggy to automobile, from slide rule to personal computer, from log cabin to skyscraper. But they can function only insofar as they are free. Businessmen (and all hard-working Americans) fare best in a market free of all regulations, in which they deal voluntarily and to mutual benefit with investors, employees and customers and in which all are governed by clear laws against force and fraud."

While it's nice to believe industries can self-regulate, too often their good intentions (and I'm giving them the benefit of the doubt, here), end up as ideas to be addressed in the future.

Let's face it. Each industry sector is most concerned, understandably, with its own self-interests, namely sales and profits. Isn't that one of the key reasons government agencies get involved with this sort of thing; to do what others avoid (except when they try to peddle their influence)? Isn't the big advantage of having government agencies responsible for the health and welfare of the American public that they can be objective and not have to look at the bottom line?

So what happens when a food industry is allowed to "self-regulate?" "It's a recipe for food poisoning," says the Food Policy Institute at the Consumer Federation of America (CFA). CFA is an association of approximately three hundred pro-consumer groups formed in 1968 to advance consumer interest though advocacy and education.

For example, take the listeria outbreak in 2002. In response to industry pressure, in 2001 the USDA initiated a program based on the notion of "voluntary regulation." After more than one hundred twenty people in seven northeastern states became ill with listeriosis and thirteen died after contracting the disease from contaminated poultry. In response to this outbreak, the poultry industry was forced to recall 27.4 million pounds of fresh and process turkey and chicken.

The poultry industry and the USDA argued that the victims got sick because they didn't act responsibly. CFA director, Carol Tucker Foreman says that's hogwash. She says the illnesses are the result of inexcusable dereliction of duty by the government agency charged with assuring meat safety. "The Bush Administration has stopped new regulations that require companies to test their products for listeria monocytogenes and permits meat and poultry companies to mislabel their products "ready-to-eat," assuring that more people will fall victim to this virulent pathogen, which kills 20 percent of those it infects."

Foreman says many of the meat and poultry products that cause listeriosis are mislabeled: "They state the products are 'cooked,' and 'ready-to-eat.' If you are pregnant or immune suppressed they are not 'ready-to-eat,' but must be reheated. The USDA should prohibit companies from misleading consumers."

But it's not just listeria. In a preliminary study, the General Accounting Office (GAO) found that five of the eleven plants in a pilot project of "self regulation," were less successful in controlling salmonella, and only one plant met the standard for eliminating visible fecal contamination. Of the eleven plants, only two had lower salmonella than under the traditional system. "This pilot project should be dumped in the garbage along with the dirty chickens it produces," says Foreman. "The only reason for the administration to go forward after the GAO report is to give in to the poultry industry's pressure to run their production lines faster. Faster line speeds result in more fecal matter on poultry. Consumers do not want poop on their poultry."

PART II

Beyond Alphabet Goop: Sorting It All Out

Now that I have probably totally spooked you—and you're convinced both the government and the food industry are conspiring against us—I have some good news. The fact is there are plenty of conscientious nutritional researchers producing terrific science. And, they're working towards improving our nutritional knowledge base. The information is out there. The trick is knowing what to look for to separate the best from the lobby-induced, politically motivated, compromised standards. That's the purpose of this next section.

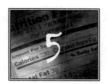

Nutritional Science Explained

No doubt our knowledge about nutrition has improved tremendously over the past one hundred years. In the United States, for example, women can expect to live thirty years longer than their ancestors of just a few short generations ago, and men—an additional twenty-five years. These gains can be attributed to advancement in scientific knowledge and techniques not only in the prevention and treatment of serious diseases, but also in the role nutrition plays in our well-being.

While scientific research obviously benefits us, the scientific process and buzz words often baffle us—not to mention thr conflicting information we hear about how good/bad something is for us to eat. We all want science to give us straight and consistent information. Unfortunately, one day an expert says one thing and the next week, a new study says the opposite. It can be frustrating—especially when you're making your best effort to live a healthy lifestyle—and can cause us to give up in frustration. Why bother making changes when today's highly recommended choice may be tomorrow's bad example?

A Couple of Perfect Examples

A classic case of such flip-flopping in nutrition is the butter vs. margarine controversy. Years ago, when research started to point toward the dangers of saturated fat for the cardiovascular system, researchers recommended people switch from butter, which is high in saturated fat, to low-saturated-fat margarine. But, further research showed margarine contained "trans fat" found to be even worse for the heart than saturated fat. While some people got the first message they didn't necessarily get the second. Those who heard both weren't sure who to believe. (Cynics figured the dairy industry was behind the resurrection of butter—and to some degree they were right.)

Another example is eating eggs. Not too many years ago, we were told eggs were good sources of protein, then we were told they were loaded with cholesterol and to limit—if not totally eliminate— eating them. Recently it was discovered eggs weren't the sole culprit; it was how we prepared them (fried in fat) and what we ate with them—often fatty bacon or sausage. So, to some degree, eggs are back in style (and the egg industry thanks you!).

But hold on just a minute. While we now know that for most people, eating eggs doesn't raise cholesterol, for a few people, eating eggs is risky. In a study of twenty-five people—granted it's a small sample—appearing in the March 2000 edition of the *Journal of the American. Dietetic Association*, the subjects ate twelve eggs a week for six weeks. For twenty-three of them, cholesterol stayed the same. But for two people, "bad" LDL cholesterol soared by 25 percent. Once again, we're not all "average."

These are excellent examples of how research often works. Scientific research is a vigorous process that often moves forward slowly—while appearing to move backwards at times. Recommendations are made based on the best science available at the time, using (hopefully) improved technology to produce new research and updated results, while revising advice. But— and this is a big but—nothing is ever 100 percent; there are always exceptions.

Fortunately, radical shifts in advice are the exception today. There's far more research on diet and health available now than in the past, and it's coming from scientists using better methods. This means that through better science, today's diet recommendations are stronger and involve much less guesswork than in the past. Plus, thanks to the mixed blessings of the Internet and TV, they're publicized better.

Granted, contradictions in research results still occur—once again partially due to the mixed blessings of advancing communications—but also because more researchers are performing studies and reporting their results. (Perhaps fulfilling the scientific imperative to publish or perish to some degree? Hmmm...)

The reality is that with many different people studying topics in many different ways, it's natural for results to differ. The key—and what should drive health recommendations—is the accumulation of the weight of evidence on a particular topic.

Here's a good analogy for the "weight" of evidence towards a particular recommendation. I wish I were clever enough to come up with it myself, but credit must go to the Harvard School of Public Health.

Harvard describes the research process as placing stones on an old-fashioned balance scale. When enough weight accumulates on one side, the scale tips in favor of a particular recommendation. And the more weight there is on one side, the stronger the recommendation is and the more evidence it would take to change it.

If, on one side of the scale, you have over forty studies showing that moderate alcohol intake can lower the risk of heart disease and, on the other, one or two studies that contradict those results, the scale would hardly budge. The weight of evidence would still be greatly in favor of moderate alcohol intake protecting against heart disease. Indeed, the link between alcohol and heart disease is so strong that it's known as an established relationship.

Unfortunately, often the weight of evidence is not as great. Sometimes, there are only a few studies tackling a particular question. In other cases, a large number of studies may lie on one side, but there may also be some particularly significant studies on the other side as well—just enough to raise doubts.

When this happens, scientists offer a caveat; they say something like, "there's a probable link" between a behavior and a disease.

There are also "possible links" where the weight of evidence is still less and, in effect, the scale only tips slightly to one side. Possible links often develop in new, emerging areas of study, where a few studies have found a relationship, but more studies need to be done to confirm the results. A high intake of trans fat and an increased risk of diabetes is an example of a possible relationship that needs to be confirmed.

In addition, the scale's likelihood of tipping reflects not only the number of stones placed on one scale, but also the size of those stones. Naturally, "heavier" stones make the scale tip faster than smaller ones. Likewise, big, well-designed studies tend to play a more important role in establishing and shaping health recommendations, than lighter, less-well-designed studies.

Types of Studies

Large studies following human participants over a period of time—known as randomized trials and cohort studies—tend to provide more reliable results than smaller studies that ask people about their past activities, which are called case-control studies.

There are many different types of research studies, and each has distinct strengths and weaknesses. In general, randomized trials and cohort studies provide the best information when looking at the link between a certain factor—such as diet—and a health outcome—heart disease, for example.

Laboratory and Animal Studies

These are studies done in laboratories on cells, tissue or animals. Laboratories provide strictly controlled conditions and are often the genesis of scientific ideas that go on to have a broad impact on human health. However, laboratory studies are only a starting point, since animals or cells are no substitute for humans.

Case-control Studies

These studies look at the characteristics of one group of people who already have a certain health outcome (the cases) and compare them to a similar group of people who do not have the outcome (the controls). While case-control studies can be done quickly and relatively cheaply, they aren't ideal for studying diet because they gather information from the past. People with illnesses often recall past behaviors differently from those without illness. This opens such studies to potential inaccuracy and bias in the information they gather.

Cohort Studies

These studies follow large groups of people over a long period of time. Researchers regularly gather information from the people in the study on a wide variety of variables (like meat intake, physical activity level and weight). Once a specified amount of time has elapsed, the characteristics of people in the group are compared to test specific hypotheses (like the link between carotenoids and glaucoma or meat intake and prostate cancer).

Though time-consuming and expensive, cohort studies generally provide more reliable information than case-control studies because they don't rely on information from the past. Cohort studies gather the information all along and before anyone develops the disease being studied. As a group, these types of studies have provided valuable information about the link between lifestyle factors and disease.

Randomized Trials

Like cohort studies, these studies follow a group of people over time. However, with randomized trials, the researchers actually intervene to see how a specific behavior change or treatment, for example, affects a health outcome. They are called "randomized trials" because people in the study are randomly assigned either to receive or not receive the intervention. This randomization helps researchers hone in on the true effect the intervention has on the health outcome. However, randomized trials also have drawbacks, especially when it comes to diet. While they are good at looking at topics like vitamin supplements and cancer, when the change in diet is more involved than say taking a vitamin pill, participants begin to have trouble keeping to their prescribed diets. Such involved interventions can also become very expensive.

Sound Science Follows, It Doesn't Lead

While they might have a pretty good idea, good scientists, grounded in sound principles, never exactly know where their research will lead them. Conclusions that once seemed logical and fairly solid may be revised—or completely overturned—as more and better research is done on a particular topic.

Take, for example, the relationship between fiber and colon cancer. Years ago, a high fiber intake was regularly recommended as one way to lower the risk for colon cancer. This advice was based on studies in countries showing people who had high fiber intakes tended to have lower rates of colon cancer than the rates found in countries where the people ate less fiber. But this didn't tell the whole story.

While they are often good points to start, "descriptive" studies generally can't address all of the factors that might account for differences in rates of disease. While fiber intake could indeed have something to do with the differences in colon cancer rates, the differences could also involve many other things that differ between countries, including other diet or lifestyle factors. When studies that can take such things into account on an individual level began to look at the issue of fiber and colon cancer, the picture became much less clear. In fact, a number of case-control studies found that a high fiber intake was linked to a lower risk of colon cancer, but many did not.

Given these wavering results—and because case-control studies are not an optimal way to assess food intake (since they rely on participants' recollections of what they ate in the past), more research using better methods was needed.

That didn't mean health professionals didn't recommend a high fiber intake for people trying to lower their risk of colon cancer. Better to be safe than sorry. Not until the results of cohort studies came out did this recommendation begin to lose its backing.

Because cohort studies observe a group of people over time, their findings are generally stronger than those of case-control studies, especially when it comes to something like diet and colon cancer. What most of these cohort studies found was that fiber intake had very little, if any, link with colon cancer.

Findings such as these were further bolstered by the results of randomized trials—which many consider the best research tool.

These studies took a group of people and randomly assigned individuals to one of two groups. One group was put on a high-fiber diet, while the other group followed a lower-fiber diet. After three or four years, the two groups were compared and no difference was found in rates of colon polyps—noncancerous growths that can turn into cancer. While realizing colon polyps are not cancer (but knowing that it's believed all colon cancers start as polyps), researchers saw it as strong evidence that fiber intake has no direct link with colon cancer.

In this case, the path of discovery led from widespread belief in a clear link between fiber and colon cancer to acceptance of the likelihood that there was no strong link between the two. In other words, sound investigative techniques kept researchers from "drawing conclusions" prematurely. What started out as a clear connection based on findings from broad, descriptive studies, eventually unraveled as more and better-quality research unveiled the actual nature of the relationship. It's an excellent example of how research can often develop when scientists don't "push" the results.

But keep one thing in mind; even a weak relationship is difficult to exclude altogether. Further studies might yet demonstrate some effect of fiber on colon cancer, although such a finding wouldn't alter the conclusion that other means must be sought to prevent colon cancer.

Is the Media to Blame?

The media knows people are intrigued by scientific discoveries, especially if it has to do with their health. While true science can be a slow, deliberate process, the news media outlets relish opportunities to be the first to trumpet new discoveries—even if the announcement is premature. And it's the media reports on health that are responsible for much of the frustration the public feels toward the public health community.

With their emphasis on short, "newsworthy" pieces with great visual elements and sound bites, the media often only report the results of single studies, and many stories are chosen simply because the results run contrary to current health recommendations. Because such reports provide little information about how the new results fit in with other evidence on the topic, the public is left to assume that, once again, the scientists screwed up and are now backtracking.

Questions to Ask

Fortunately, in many cases it only takes a few incisive questions to get at the heart of a research-related news story and see how important the results are for you personally. One of the most crucial things to keep in mind is the issue we've already discussed above: how a given study fits into the entire body of evidence on a topic. Whenever reading or watching a news story on health, try to glean answers to the following ten questions:

1. Who conducted the research? Was it a reputable university or health organization?
2. Where was it conducted? Was it in the U.S. or in another country? Dietary habits can differ between nations and cultures.
3. Who funded the research?
4. Does the study appear, or is it scheduled to appear, in a reputable medical journal? (Journals such as *Lancet*, *New England Journal of Medicine*, *JAMA* or ones published by specific disease foundations are most reliable.)
5. Was the study based on clinical data or through medical records?
6. If through medical records, how far back do the records go? Eating habits (as well as other factors such as pollution and lifestyle) have changed over time. Results based on habits from the 1940s might not be relevant today.
7. Are they simply reporting the results of a single study? If so, where does it fit in with other studies on the topic? Rarely is a single study conclusive enough to warrant people to change their behaviors.
8. How large is the study? Usually, the more subjects involved the more reliable the results—assuming the researchers used sound scientific techniques.
9. Were the study subjects animals or humans? While there are merits to using mice, rats, monkeys and other animals, they are not people. To test a nutritional theory from animal research, there should be additional research conducted on humans. Despite what you might observe at raucous sporting events—or if you

commute to work on a congested highway—people are not animals.

10. Did the study look at real disease endpoints, like cancer or heart disease or symptoms believed to lead to a disease? Chronic diseases typically can take years to develop. To speed up the process, researchers sometimes look at markers for these diseases, like narrowing of the arteries for heart disease or bone density for osteoporosis. While they're good clues, they don't always develop into the disease.

Here's an important bonus question to which you need to know the answer:

11. Who's reporting the results? Is the data and recommendations coming from the CDC, National Institute of Health, a reputable university or foundation, such as the American Cancer Society? Or is it coming from a lobby group or other organization with its own agenda?

Hopefully, these tips and examples will help you discern accurate news from rumors and preliminary results. While the facts based on well-thought-out scientific investigation might not be sexy enough to lead the 6 o'clock news, with a little knowledge and a little scrutiny on your part, you should be able to separate fact from preliminary findings and half-baked fantasy.

Now it's time to move on and look at the things that come packaged in our foods; the individual nutrients we need—along with the things we don't.

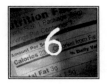

Eating 101

Besides breathing, the one thing we'll all probably do today is eat food. Everything we eat contains one or more of these seven basic components:

- proteins
- fats
- carbohydrates (simple and complex)
- fiber (a component of some carbohydrates)
- water
- vitamins
- minerals

To benefit from these nutrients, food must be digested and distributed—or excreted—to keep our bodies functioning properly.

The first three—carbohydrates, protein and fat—are known as macronutrients. All of the foods you eat are composed of these three. Some foods are primarily carbohydrates, others are mainly proteins, and others are mostly fats. Other foods are combinations of two or all three. A slice of pizza is a perfect example. The crust and tomato sauce provide the carbohydrates, and the cheese provides protein and fat.

To meet the body's daily energy and nutritional needs, the latest nutritional standards from the National Academy of Sciences recommends adults get 45 percent to 65 percent of their calories from carbohydrates, 20 percent to 35 percent from fat, and 10 percent to 35 percent from protein. Earlier guidelines called for diets with 50 percent or more of carbohydrates and 30 percent or less of fat; protein intake recommendations are the same. The newest recommendations for children are similar to those for adults, except that infants and younger children need a slightly higher proportion of fat—25 percent to 40 percent of their caloric intake.

I've included the others items—fiber, water, vitamins and minerals—since they also are critical components of what we eat and drink. All but vitamins and minerals are covered in this chapter.

You'll notice artificial coloring, flavorings, pesticides, and the like aren't on the list and don't belong to any of these groups. Those are just extra goodies food manufacturers add to increase crop yield, extend shelf life and make food look prettier. None of them are beneficial to your health and well-being.

Here are small sketches of the first five food elements. Longer, more detailed descriptions follow later in this chapter.

Protein

Protein makes up the greatest portion of our body weight and is involved in most of the chemical process within the body. Proteins are the building blocks of muscles, ligaments, tendons, organs, glands, nails, hair, body fluids, enzymes, hormones and genes.

Amino acids are formed when protein is broken down by digestion. Of the twenty-two amino acids, eight are essential—meaning they cannot be manufactured by the body and must come from our food. The rest are nonessential, meaning they can be manufactured by the body—with proper nutrition.

Fat

Fat is required in your diet for your body to function properly but, too much fat can have a negative impact on your health. Fat is a good source of energy. It contains twice as many calories per gram as carbohydrates or proteins. Saturated and trans fats increase the risk of coronary artery disease by raising blood cholesterol levels. High blood levels of cholesterol can lead to a narrowing of the arteries and an increased risk of heart attack and stroke. Polyunsaturated fats lower blood cholesterol but also seem susceptible to oxidation. Oxidation is a process that enables cells in the arteries to absorb fats and cholesterol. Over time, oxidation speeds the buildup of plaques, which narrow arteries.

Certain vitamins are fat soluble. The only way to get these vitamins is to eat fat. In the same way that there are essential amino acids, there are essential fatty acids (for example, linoleic acid is used to build cell membranes). You must obtain these fatty acids from food you eat because your body has no way to make them.

Carbohydrates

There are two types of carbohydrates that give the body energy: simple and complex. The body breaks down carbohydrates into a sugar known as glucose. Glucose is the only sugar that our brain can use as fuel, and it gets stored in the muscles as reserved energy. But the same sugar turns into fat if you have too much of it. Simple carbohydrates convert easily into glucose while the complex types take more time to convert and move more slowly into the body, so they don't increase your blood sugar as quickly. It is the complex carbohydrates that are good for you as they have vitamins, minerals and fiber.

Fiber

Fiber is a carbohydrate, a large group of widely different compounds, and is a part of plants that cannot be digested by enzymes in the human intestinal tract. Cellulose is the most important compound of fiber. It assists in the digestive process, although it cannot be digested. Fiber prevents constipation and related disorders such as hemorrhoids. Fiber helps lower blood cholesterol.

Water

We cannot survive for long without water because 60 to 70 percent of our body weight consists of water as every cell in the body and 90 percent of our blood contains water. Water is needed to digest food and transport nutrients, to build and repair tissues, and to eliminate waste and regulate body temperature. Water actually suppresses appetite naturally and helps the body to metabolize stored fat.

Studies show that a decrease in water intake will cause fat deposits to increase, while an increase in water intake actually reduces fat deposits—leading to fat loss. Water also helps the liver convert triglycerides (fats) into usable energy. Kidneys also need water to function properly.

New Guidelines

In September, 2002, the National Academy of Sciences (NAS) issued a new report, altering previous guidelines about fat consumption. The NAS urged people to include more fiber in their diet and to cut back on foods with added sugar, including soft drinks, candy and pastries.

To meet the body's daily energy and nutritional needs while minimizing the risk for chronic disease, the new report recommends adults receive 20 percent to 35 percent of their calories from fat and 10 percent to 35 percent from protein.

The voluminous report also sets broad new targets for how many calories to eat daily, based in part on physical activity. The report also establishes the first recommended dietary allowance for carbohydrates. The NAS recommended doubling the amount of exercise Americans should have daily. It sets a daily goal of sixty minutes a day of moderate intensity exercise—twice the amount recommended by the U.S. Surgeon General in 1996.

The 2002 nutritional recommendations recommend adults and children consume at least 130 grams a day of carbohydrates—something, the report notes, the vast majority of Americans already achieve. It also establishes the first recommended intake for two healthy fats that appear to help reduce sudden death from heart disease.

Known as polyunsaturated fats, these beneficial fats can't be manufactured by the body, so they need to be eaten every day. Food sources include milk and flaxseed, soybean, safflower and corn oils. At the same time, the report underscores the health dangers of saturated fat—such as those found in fatty cuts of meat and whole-fat dairy products—and of trans fatty acids, fats often found in hardened forms of shortening used in baked goods and fried food. Dietary cholesterol, the report notes, should also be eaten sparingly, since the body naturally makes all that it needs. All three of these fats help contribute to the risk of heart disease, the report notes.

Issued by the NAS after more than two years of study, the new Dietary Reference Intakes (DRIs), also set a broader range for fat and carbohydrate intake for healthy people. Echoing the National Heart, Lung and Blood Institute's guidelines, the report said that healthy diets can include as much as 35 percent fat—or about 5 percent more than has been previously recommended. The report also notes, however, that fat intake can safely drop as low as 20 percent of daily calories. Most important is for Americans to reach a healthy weight and maintain it.

As should be obvious to us all, more than half of Americans are overweight or obese. Childhood obesity is also increasing, and with it, the incidence of health problems once seen only in adults, including type II diabetes. For this reason, the new recommendations emphasize that it's not just what you eat that's important but how many calories you burn each day.

The National Academies' Institute of Medicine published a new DRI report in September 2002 saying people can consume up to 25 percent of their diets in added sugars. That doesn't sound right to a lot of people, and health-conscious eaters can easily get confused about what the new guidelines mean. It's actually okay to eat added sugars as 25 percent of your diet?

Rachel Johnson, Ph.D., R.D., professor of nutrition and acting dean of the University of Vermont's College of Agriculture and Life Science, contributed the guidelines on sugar to the Institute of Medicine's report. Here she clarifies the numbers and the intention of the report. "It's not a recommendation to eat 25 percent of calories as added sugars, that's an absolute ceiling," says Johnson.

For example, at 25 percent of calories from added sugars, intake of key vitamins and nutrients significantly decreases to adversely affect health. Eating added sugars also either adds calories or dilutes important nutrients. Not all foods containing added sugars are equal. Some sweets come with vitamins, fiber and other beneficial nutrients. Stick with the treats that include at least a few useful nutrients like granola bars or dried fruit snacks. Sweets like chocolate, soda pop, and hard candies, to name a few, just aren't worth it.

Metabolism: How Our Bodies Use Energy

While this is not a book about dieting, maintaining a healthy weight is critical to overall well-being. Here is some basic background you should know.

You might know metabolism is linked to your weight, but you probably don't know how important metabolism is and how it works. Some aspects of your metabolism you can control, and others you can't. Here's a basic primer on metabolism.

Simply, metabolism is a biochemical process. It combines nutrients with oxygen to release the energy your body needs to function.

There are two phases to metabolism, anabolic and catabolic. The anabolic, or constructive, phase converts compounds from nutrients into substances the body can use. The catabolic, or destructive, phase reconverts the substances into simpler compounds to get the energy release needed to keep body cells going.

Metabolism is measured in calories. The number of calories you burn in a day depends on several factors, including your basal metabolic rate (BMR), how often you exercise and your body's muscle-to-fat ratio.

If you have a fever, your metabolism can increase by 10 to 30 percent. If you're a woman and still menstruating, your metabolic rate is slightly higher just before your period than at any other time in your cycle, which might help explain the frequent urges women have to snack during that time. Digesting food causes the metabolism to speed up temporarily. Hormones, such as insulin, also can affect your metabolism.

Here the simple facts. One pound equals 3,500 calories. To lose one pound of weight you must burn calories through physical activity and reduce the number of calories you eat for a total of 3,500.

Basal Metabolic Rate

Your BMR refers to how many calories you burn at rest to maintain vital body functions, including brain activity, heartbeat and breathing. It usually accounts for half or more of the calories you expend daily. Your abdominal tissues alone account for about 27 percent of your BMR, largely to manufacture compounds your body needs to function normally.

The more lean muscle mass you have in your body, the more calories you tend to burn. That's one of the reasons experts tout strength training as a way to build lean muscle mass. It's also why men, who tend to have more lean muscle than women and, therefore, burn more calories, have the ability to lose weight faster than women.

As you age, BMR decreases at a rate of about 2 percent a decade. That's why it gets harder to control your weight as you get older. But the reason your BMR declines has more to do with losing muscle mass than it does with aging. If you work to maintain your muscle through exercise, then you can keep your metabolism from slowing so much.

You use about 10 percent of the calories you consume to digest your food. It's known as the thermic effect of food. So, if you eat 1,800 calories in any given day, you'll burn about 180 of them simply digesting, absorbing and metabolizing nutrients.

Depending on how much you exercise, you expend between 15 percent and 40 percent of your caloric intake on physical activity. But remember, it's not just strenuous exercise—but all activity—that helps boost your calorie burn. That includes taking the stairs instead of the elevator and getting up to change the TV channel. It all adds up.

If you have tried to lose weight, you may have convinced yourself that it's so difficult because your metabolism is slow. One way to know for sure is to have your doctor test your metabolism. But don't be surprised if you find out your rate is normal. "For 90-plus percent of the people we test who think they have low metabolism, it's pretty normal," says Michael Jensen, M.D., an endocrinologist at Mayo Clinic in Rochester, MN. "It's actually only a tiny fraction of people who burn fewer calories at rest than they should according to their height, weight and age."

Often the problem is perception. "If you're having difficulty losing weight or are gaining weight easily, we have to look at what are realistic expectations for the rate of weight loss," Jensen says. "Popular magazines give the impression that you can lose 10 to 20 pounds a month. People who lose weight that fast typically are losing huge amounts of water and lean muscle. For most women, even if you cut their food intake by 25 percent, which is a lot, they'd lose only a pound of fat a week."

Although you've probably heard of the dangers of yo-yo dieting, Dr. Jensen says chronic dieting probably has little permanent effect on your metabolism. However, taking in fewer calories means that you have less energy to burn. "When you diet intensely, you move around less," he says, "You get a little sluggish." So what's a woman to do? "Get more physically active," Jensen says. "Take a walk, ride a bike. Don't take all the shortcuts. Do everything you can throughout the day to get extra steps in."

Now that you know how your metabolism works, you know you have some control over it. Keep the metabolic fires burning by keeping your body fat down and your muscle up. And don't forget, every step you take burns more calories.

Calculating Your Resting Metabolism

You can get an approximate measure of your basal metabolism, the amount of energy your body uses at rest, with the following formula. (Unless you're a whiz at doing math in your head, use a calculator.)

- 655 + (9.6 X weight in kilograms) + (1.8 X height in centimeters) - (4.7 X age) = BMR
- To convert pounds to kilograms, divide your weight by 2.2.
- To convert inches to centimeters, multiply your height in inches by 2.54.

So, if you're a fifty-year-old, 5-foot, 5-inch woman who weighs 150 pounds, your formula would look like this:

$$655 + (9.6 \times 68.18) + (1.7 \times 165.1) - (4.7 \times 50) = 655 + 654.5 + 280.67 - 235 = 1{,}355 \text{ calories}$$

Calories

The September 2002 RDA/DRI report recommends total calories to be consumed by individuals of given heights, weights, and genders for each of four different levels of physical activity. For example, a thirty-year-old woman who is 5 feet, 5 inches tall and weighs 111 to 150 pounds should consume between 1,800 and 2,000 calories daily if she lives a sedentary lifestyle.

However, if she is a very active person, her recommended total caloric intake increases from 2,500 to 2,800 calories per day. If her lifestyle fits the moderately active category as defined in the report, which is the minimum level of activity to decrease risk of chronic disease, she should eat between 2,200 and 2,500 calories daily. Using grams for the recommended ranges of intake, she should consume 55 to 97 grams of fat and 285 to 375 grams of carbohydrates per day. The report stresses the importance of balancing diet with exercise.

Confused? I hope not. The next chapter includes greater details about each food component, and how they can help or hinder our health.

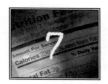

Our Real Needs for Macronutrients

As I stated in the previous chapter, everything we eat contains one or more of seven basic components:

- proteins
- fats
- carbohydrates (simple and complex)
- fiber (a component of some carbohydrates)
- water
- vitamins
- minerals

The rest of this chapter will discuss what role each of these groups plays in providing the body with the building blocks necessary for good health.

Our Real Needs for Protein

What is protein? With so much emphasis lately on carbohydrates and fat, protein often becomes an afterthought. Too bad, since it is vitally important. Lack of protein can cause growth failure, loss of muscle mass, decreased immunity, weakening of the heart and respiratory system, and death.

Adults need a daily minimum of about 8 grams of protein for about every 20 pounds of weight per day to maintain tissue. In the United States and other developed countries, it's easy to get the minimum daily requirement of protein. Beyond that, there's relatively little solid information on the ideal amount of protein in the diet, a healthy target for calories contributed by protein, or the best kinds of protein.

As I stated in the previous chapter, amino acids are formed when protein is broken down by digestion. Amino acids are the most important, powerful and significant nutrients we can consume, with 75 percent of our dry body weight (minus water) made up of amino acids. By comparison, vitamins and minerals account for 1.5 percent of dry body weight.

Amino Acids

Amino acids offer a myriad of health benefits. Aminos build cells and repair tissue; they form antibodies to combat invading bacteria and viruses and are a vital part of the enzyme and hormonal system. They build nucleoproteins (RNA & DNA) and participate in every chemical reaction in the body including carrying oxygen throughout the body and participating in muscle activity.

All amino acids, except one, are neurotransmitters. Also, 95 percent of hormones are amino acids.

While it's clear too little protein is clearly a problem, what about too much? The digestion of protein releases acids that the body usually neutralizes with calcium and other buffering agents in the blood. Eating lots of protein—as recommended in popular no-carb diets—requires lots of calcium. Some calcium can end up coming from bones. Following a high-protein diet for a few weeks probably won't have much effect on bone strength but doing it for a long time, might.

In the landmark Nurses' Health Study at Harvard, researchers found women who ate more than 95 grams of protein a day were 20 percent more likely to have broken a wrist over a twelve-year period than those eating an average amount of protein (less than 68 grams a day).

Types of Protein

Some proteins contain all the amino acids needed to construct new proteins. This kind is called complete protein. Animal sources of protein tend to be complete. Other protein lacks one or more amino acids that the body can't make from scratch or create by modifying another amino acid. Called incomplete proteins, these usually come from fruits, vegetables, grains and nuts.

Vegetarians need to be aware of this difference. To get all the amino acids needed to make new protein (and thus to keep the body's systems in good shape) people who don't eat meat, fish, poultry, eggs or dairy products should eat a variety of protein-containing foods each day.

Animal protein and vegetable protein probably have the same effects on health. It's how the protein is served that can make a difference. A 6-ounce broiled Porterhouse steak delivers 38 grams of protein, but also has 44 grams of fat—more than a third of the grams as saturated fat. That's almost three-fourths of the recommended daily intake for saturated fat. Eating the same amount of salmon, on the other hand, provides 34 grams of protein and 18 grams of fat—only 4 of them saturated. Even better, a cup of cooked lentils also has 34 grams of protein, but less than 1 gram of fat.

To get the protein you need, fish or poultry are better then steaks. If you must have beef, select the leanest cuts. Even better options are vegetable sources of protein, such as beans, nuts and whole grains.

Protein and Chronic Disease

The most solid connection between proteins and health has to do with a common disorder of the immune system. Proteins in food and in the environment are responsible for a variety of allergies. Allergies are basically overreactions of the immune system to what should be harmless proteins. Beyond that, relatively little evidence has been gathered regarding the effect of proteins on the development of chronic diseases.

Here's what preliminary research shows:

Cardiovascular disease. There's been only one large study investigating the association between dietary protein and heart disease or stroke. In the Nurses' Health Study, women who ate the most protein (about 110 grams per day) were 25 percent less likely to have a heart attack or to have died of heart disease than the women who ate the least protein (about 68 grams per day) over a fourteen-year period. Whether the protein came from animals or vegetables, or whether it was part of low-fat or higher-fat diets didn't seem to matter. These results offer reassurance that eating a lot of protein doesn't harm the heart. In fact, it is possible that eating more protein while cutting back on easily digested carbohydrates might benefit the heart.

Diabetes. Proteins found in cow's milk may play a role in the development of type I diabetes (formerly called juvenile or insulin-dependent diabetes). That's one reason why cow's milk isn't recommended for infants. Later in life, the amount of protein in the diet doesn't seem to adversely affect the development of type II diabetes, although research in this area is ongoing.

Cancer. There's no good evidence that eating a little protein, or a lot of it, influences cancer risk.

Protein and Weight Control

In short-term studies, a lower-calorie diet that includes more protein and fewer carbohydrates is more effective for losing weight or keeping weight steady than a lower-calorie, high-carbohydrate diet. Eating high-protein foods such as beef, chicken, fish, or beans makes you feel full for longer because they slow the movement of food from the stomach to the intestine. This strategy may also delay hunger signals. Compared with carbohydrates, the digestion of protein causes smaller, steadier increases in blood sugar. This helps avoid the steep climbs and quick drops in blood sugar that occur after eating rapidly digested carbohydrates. Unfortunately, few data have been collected on the longer-term effects of a high-protein diet on weight control.

Say "Soy"

Soybeans have been getting a lot of attention lately. Some research suggests the possibility that regularly eating soybeans or soy-based foods can lower cholesterol, "chill" hot flashes, prevent breast and prostate cancer, aid weight loss, and ward off osteoporosis. These effects may be due to a unique characteristic of soybeans: their high concentrations of isoflavones, a type of plant-made estrogen.

This research has prompted scads of media reports touting the joys of soy. It also has food makers churning out new soy products that are beginning to move into the mainstream. As is so often the case, though, many of the claims made for soy go far beyond the available evidence:

Heart disease. There's decent evidence that soy lowers cholesterol levels. A 1995 meta-analysis of thirty-eight controlled clinical trials showed that eating approximately 50 grams of soy protein a day in place of animal protein reduced total cholesterol levels by 9.3 percent, LDL cholesterol by 12.9 percent, and triglycerides by 10.5 percent. Such reductions, if sustained over time, could mean a 20 percent reduction in the risk of myocardial infarction or other forms of cardiovascular disease. Individuals with very high cholesterol levels in the vicinity of 300 mg/dL appeared to benefit most from eating soy-based foods. Keep in mind that 50 grams of soy protein is the equivalent of 1 pound of tofu or eight 8-ounce glasses of soy milk a day. The American Heart Association now recommends including soy-based foods as part of a heart-healthy diet.

Hot flashes. Soy has also been investigated as a treatment for hot flashes and other problems that often accompany menopause. In theory, this makes sense. Soybeans are rich in plant estrogens, also called phytoestrogens. In some tissues, these substances mimic the action of estrogen. So they could cool hot flashes by giving a woman an estrogen-like boost during a time of dwindling estrogen levels. Yet carefully controlled studies haven't demonstrated a clear benefit for soy.

Breast cancer. In some tissues, phytoestrogens block the action of estrogen. If this occurs in breast tissue, for example, then eating soy could reduce the risk of breast cancer because estrogen stimulates the growth and multiplication of breast and breast cancer cells. However, studies to date haven't provided a clear answer, with some showing a benefit and others showing no association between soy consumption and breast cancer. Large prospective studies now underway should offer better information regarding soy and breast cancer risk.

Obviously, soy isn't the wonder food many claim it to be. Unsettling reports suggest that concentrated supplements of soy proteins may stimulate the growth of breast cancer cells. Too much soy could also lead to memory problems. Among older women of Japanese ancestry living in Hawaii, those who relied on the traditional soy-based diet were more likely to have cognitive problems than those who switched to a more Western diet. These preliminary findings suggest that too much anti-estrogen in the wrong place at the wrong time could be harmful.

Still, the U.S. Food and Drug Administration now allows food makers to claim on the label of low-fat foods containing at least 6.25 grams of soy protein that soy can help reduce the risk of heart disease.

Consider Other Legumes

Legumes—which are high in protein—refer to a large family of plants whose seeds develop inside pods and are usually dried for ease of storage. Legumes include beans, peas and lentils.

You should be able to find these common legumes in your supermarket:

- white or navy beans
- lima beans
- pinto and black beans
- black-eyed peas
- split peas
- brown lentils

Try shopping in ethnic markets for less common legumes. Indian markets, for example, usually offer a good selection of lentils, including pink- and orange-colored ones. Chickpeas are readily found in Italian delicatessens, where they are more likely labeled garbanzo beans. Buying legumes in bulk often provides the freshest product at the greatest savings.

You should buy recently dried legumes. Whether buying bulk or packaged legumes, get them from a source with a quick turnover, so you can be fairly certain they're fresh. Newly dried legumes cook more quickly. Look for legumes of a uniform size that will cook evenly. Be sure they are free of mold or any other impurities.

Consider these ways to incorporate legumes into everyday meals:

* Feature beans, peas or lentils in soups, stews, casseroles and salads.
* Try tofu in place of meat in stir-fries.
* Use puréed beans as the basis for dips and spreads.

Storing legumes. Store legumes at room temperature. After purchase, place in tightly covered jars away from heat, light and moisture. They'll keep well for up to one year.

Cooking legumes. Carefully sort legumes before use. Bags of legumes may include a few small stones or fibers that you need to remove, along with any misshapen or discolored items, before cooking.

Pre-soak large dried legumes before cooking. Beans and other large dried legumes such as chickpeas and black-eyed peas require pre-soaking, a step that rehydrates them for more even cooking. Once soaked, the beans are ready to cook. Split peas and lentils require no pre-soaking.

For convenience, use canned legumes. Already prepared legumes are fine in dishes that don't require long simmering. Rinse them well to reduce the sodium that may have been added during processing.

Recommendations for Eating Protein

1. Get a good mix of proteins. Almost any reasonable diet will give you enough protein each day. Eating a variety of foods will ensure that you get all of the amino acids you need.

2. Pay attention to the protein package. You rarely eat straight protein. Some comes packaged with lots of unhealthy fat, like when you eat marbled beef or drink whole milk. If you eat meat, steer yourself toward the leanest cuts. If you like dairy products, skim or low-fat versions are healthier choices. Beans, soy, nuts, and whole grains offer protein without much saturated fat and with plenty of healthful fiber and micronutrients.

3. *Balance carbohydrates and protein.* Cutting back on highly processed carbohydrates—covered in the next section—and increasing protein improves levels of blood triglycerides and HDL, and so may reduce your chances of having a heart attack, stroke, or other forms of cardiovascular disease. It may also make you feel full longer, and stave off hunger pangs. Too much protein, though, could weaken bones.

4. *Eat soy in moderation.* Soybeans, tofu, and other soy-based foods are an excellent alternative to red meat. Two to four servings a week is a good target. And stay away from supplements that contain concentrated soy protein or soy extracts, such as isoflavones. Larger amounts of soy may soothe hot flashes and other menopause-associated problems, but the evidence for this is weak.

5. *Try other legumes.* These plant foods—including a variety of beans and peas—make an excellent substitute for animal sources of protein.

Our Real Needs for Fat

Fat-free, nonfat, low-fat, reduced-fat, light, zero-fat; from cereal and soup to nuts, food products today are branded with a dizzying array of fat qualifiers—to keep our fat intake low. After all, haven't we been told we must eat a low-fat, low-cholesterol diet to ward off disease and obesity? Most of the advice is not just nonsense; it's dangerous.

Current research shows the total amount of fat in the diet, whether high or low, has no real link with disease. Frankly, we *need* fat in our diets. Instead, what really matters is the type of fat in the diet. We now know there are bad fats that increase the risk for certain diseases and good fats that lower the risk. The key to sound nutrition is to substitute good fats for bad fats; especially harmful trans fats.

Also, while it's true that dietary cholesterol is linked to heart disease, it isn't the masked villain we've been led to believe it is. What should concern us is cholesterol circulating in our blood. High blood cholesterol levels greatly increase the risk for heart disease. And contrary to what may seem logical, the amount of cholesterol in food has only a small link with cholesterol levels in the blood.

The biggest influence on blood cholesterol levels is the types of fats in the diet. When there's a buildup of cholesterol in the coronary arteries—the arteries that feed the heart—the arteries are narrowed and blood flow to the heart is slowed down or blocked. With less blood, the heart gets less oxygen. When there is not enough oxygen to the heart, there may be chest pain. This is called arteriosclerosis or hardening of the arteries. The area of cholesterol buildup—called plaque—can rupture, causing a heart attack or death. Cholesterol buildup is the most common cause of heart disease. Fortunately, this buildup can be slowed or possibly even reduced.

What Is Cholesterol?

Cholesterol is a wax-like substance made in the liver of human and animals. Despite what you might think, cholesterol plays an essential role in the formation of cell membranes, some hormones, and vitamin D. Cholesterol travels between the liver and other parts of the body via the blood stream with the help of carriers called lipoproteins. Lipoproteins play a very important role in the link between blood cholesterol and heart disease.

There are two main types of lipoprotein carriers, and they essentially work in opposite directions:

Low-density lipoproteins (LDL) carry cholesterol from the liver to the rest of the body. When there is too much LDL-cholesterol in the blood, it can be deposited on the walls of the coronary arteries. Because of this, LDL-cholesterol is often referred to as the "bad" cholesterol.

High-density lipoproteins (HDL) carry cholesterol from the blood back to the liver where it is processed and eliminated from the body. HDLs make the excess cholesterol in the blood less likely to be deposited in the coronary arteries and is the reason HDL-cholesterol is often referred to as the "good" cholesterol.

When you have your cholesterol checked, the results usually show total blood cholesterol levels as well as separate counts for HDL- and LDL-cholesterol levels. In general, the higher your HDL count and the lower the LDL count, the lower your risk of arteriosclerosis and heart disease. The most recent federal guidelines from the National Cholesterol Education Program recommend the following for adults aged twenty years or older:

- Total cholesterol less than 200 mg per deciliter (mg/dl)
- HDL-cholesterol levels greater than 40 mg/dl
- LDL-cholesterol levels less than 100 mg/dl

Blood Cholesterol Levels

As I've already said, one of the most important determinants of blood cholesterol level is not total fat, but the specific types of fat. Research shows that some types of fat are clearly good for blood cholesterol and others are clearly bad. As for cholesterol in food, it does affect blood cholesterol levels but not nearly as much as many people believe.

An individual's serum cholesterol level is determined by a combination of genetic factors and diet. For some people, levels of blood cholesterol can be traced to the amount of cholesterol in their food. For others, the amount of cholesterol they eat has relatively little impact on the amount of cholesterol that circulates in the blood.

What About Cholesterol and Eggs?

Long condemned by scientists and doctors for their high cholesterol content, eggs are now making something of a comeback. In the Harvard study of over eighty thousand female nurses, researchers found that increasing cholesterol intake by 200 mg for every 1,000 calories in the diet—the equivalent of about 1.5 eggs per day for the average woman—did not appreciably increase the risk of heart disease. While it's true that egg yolks have a lot of cholesterol—and, therefore, may slightly affect blood cholesterol levels—eggs also contain nutrients that may help lower the risk of heart disease, including protein, vitamins B12 and D, riboflavin, and folate. Eating eggs in moderation can, therefore, be included as part of a healthy diet. People with diabetes, though, should probably limit themselves to only two or three eggs a week, as the study found that an egg a day may increase heart disease risk in these individuals. Those who have difficulty controlling their blood cholesterol may also want to be cautious about egg yolk intake, choosing instead egg white based foods.

The Bad Fats

These types of fats tend to negatively affect blood cholesterol levels:

Saturated fats. These are mainly animal fats. They are found in meat, seafood, whole-milk dairy products (cheese, milk, and ice cream), poultry with skin, and egg yolks. Some plant foods are also high in saturated fats and include coconut and coconut oil, palm and palm kernel oil. While saturated fats raise total blood cholesterol levels more so than dietary cholesterol, they tend to raise both the "good" HDL cholesterol as well as the "bad" LDL cholesterol.

Trans fats. Also known as trans fatty acids, these fats are produced by heating liquid vegetable oils in the presence of hydrogen—a process known as hydrogenation, which increases the shelf life of processed foods containing these oils. The more hydrogenated an oil, the harder it will be at room temperature. For example, spreadable tub margarines are less hydrogenated—meaning they have less trans fats—than a stick margarine.

Most of the trans fats found in the American diet comes from commercially prepared baked goods such as crackers, cookies and other snack foods, margarines, and processed foods. Fast foods are another common source of trans fats. French fries, onion rings, fried fish and chicken sandwiches, chicken nuggets, and doughnuts and deep-fried foods can deliver unhealthy doses of trans fats.

Trans fats are worse for cholesterol levels than saturated fats because they raise the "bad" LDL-cholesterol while also lowering "good" HDL-cholesterol.

The Good Fats

The good fats—known as unsaturated fats—tend to improve blood cholesterol levels. There are two kinds of unsaturated fats, polyunsaturated and monounsaturated. Both come mainly from plant sources.

- *Polyunsaturated fats.* These are found largely in sunflower, corn, and soybean oils.
- *Monounsaturated fats.* These are found largely in canola, peanut, and olive oils.

Both of these fats increase the "good" HDL cholesterol and decrease the "bad" LDL cholesterol. Other excellent sources of unsaturated fats are tree nuts such as walnuts and cashews and seeds such as flax and sunflower seeds.

Fat Recommendations

The latest RDA/DRI guidelines recommend people consume 20 to 35 percent of their calories from fat to prevent disease. Many health agencies, such as the American Dietetic Association, American Diabetes Association and American Heart Association, recommend limiting fat intake to 30 percent or less. There is no evidence of an ideal amount of total fat for a healthy diet. Major studies have found no link between the percentage of calories of total fat and any important health outcome—including cancer, heart disease, or weight gain. What they have found to be important, is the type of fat in the diet—and there are clear links between the different types of dietary fats and heart disease.

Of the bad fats—saturated and trans fats—trans fats are far worse when it comes to heart disease. The Nurses' Health Study found that replacing only 30 calories (7 grams) of carbohydrates every day with 30 calories (4 grams) of trans fats nearly doubled the risk of heart disease. Saturated fats increased risk as well, but not nearly as much.

For the good fats, evidence consistently shows that a high intake of unsaturated fat (compared to saturated fats) lowers the risk of heart disease. In the same study, Harvard researchers found that replacing 80 calories of carbohydrates with 80 calories of either polyunsaturated or monounsaturated fats lowered the risk of heart disease about 30 to 40 percent.

Some Good News

For the better part of a decade, it's been known that we should avoid trans fats, but we didn't know how. Not only were they nowhere to be seen on the "Nutrition Facts" portion of food labels, but only the word *hydrogenated* indicated they were part of a food product's ingredients. Once alerted to the presence of trans fats, we could only guess the amount the product contained. The only sure way to avoid trans fats was to avoid all snack foods, crackers, and packaged bakery goods.

In July 2002, Joseph Levitt, director of the Center for Food Safety and Applied Nutrition (CFSAN), said the FDA decided to go forward with a final rule to add trans fat to nutrition labels. Fifty scientists from prominent universities signed a letter supporting the label change. They claim trans fat labeling will save lives and billions of dollars in health care costs.

According to the results of a study presented in June 2000 at an American Heart Association dietary conference on fatty acids, the lead researcher said the label change could prevent in numerous deaths from heart attacks. Kathleen M. Koehler, Ph.D., MPH, an epidemiologist at the Center for Food Safety and Applied Nutrition at the Food and Drug Administration office in Washington, D.C., said removing trans fats from all margarine would prevent approximately 6,300 heart attacks including 2,100 deaths a year. Additionally, removing trans fats from only 3 percent of breads and cakes and 15 percent of cookies and crackers would prevent an estimated 17,100 heart attacks, including 5,600 deaths, she said.

Koehler adds that the proposal would likely result in the public making dietary changes that would save an estimated $25 billion to $59 billion in healthcare costs over twenty years. That's compared to a cost of $401 million to $854 million to change the labels and reformulate products, she said.

To determine the health benefits of the label changes, the researchers estimated the expected decrease in trans fat intake. They created three possible scenarios, all of which assume food companies will remove all trans fats from margarines. Based on informal surveys, the FDA estimates that about 30 percent of margarines already on the market are free of trans fats.

The first scenario suggested that 100 percent of margarines will be free of trans fats and that the change would occur as soon as the labeling changes become effective. The second scenario is that trans fats will be eliminated not only from all margarines, but also from 1.5 percent of breads and cakes and 7.5 percent of cookies and crackers over a five-year period. The third scenario has trans fats eliminated from 3 percent of breads and cakes and 15 percent of cookies and crackers over seven years after the labeling change.

"When you change your diet, cholesterol levels can change within several weeks," Koehler said. Research shows that an individual begins to see the health benefits of those changes after about three years. So in the third scenario—in which the changes would be phased in—it would take about ten years for the full health benefits to show up on a population-wide basis.

Once in effect, the new labels will tell us the calories of trans fats that one serving of a food contains and the percentage of a daily 1,500-calorie diet that those calories constitute.

But industry groups are criticizing the FDA's efforts as misleading and lacking the necessary context to adequately educate consumers. "It's good news that the FDA is poised to require trans fats on food labels, after doing nothing for nearly a decade," said Center for Science in the Public Interest Nutrition Policy Director Margo Wootan, in a written statement. "But labels that don't list a Daily Value for trans fat would be misleading because they would give no indication of whether a number of grams is a lot or a little."

The FDA based its labeling decision on a report by the food nutrition board of the National Academy of Sciences Institute of Medicine. The academy was unable to come up with a daily value for trans fats, simultaneously noting zero consumption "would require extraordinary changes in pattern of dietary intake," said Levitt of CFSAN. Based on these findings, FDA will list only the content of trans fats by grams, rather than by percentage of daily recommended value. "We will let the trans fat daily value be kept open until the scientific foundation and the academy of recommendations are there," said Levitt.

CSPI, a consumer advocacy group, originally petitioned for the labeling amendment in 1993. They believe the best solution would be to follow the Canadian labeling model and list trans-fat content alongside saturated fat, using the existing daily value of 20 grams for saturated fat. CSPI estimates disclosing trans fats on food labels would save between 2,100 and 5,600 lives each year. But some critics say there is no need to re-label foods. "I think it's wrong to scare people about their food when the science is really poor, and I think that's what's going on here," said Steve Milloy. "Medical studies linking trans fats and heart disease are flawed," he said. "They tackle these complex diseases with very limited data," Milloy said. "They draw these broad conclusions and in the long run these conclusions turn out to be junk science."

Despite Milloy's complaints, the marketplace has begun to respond to consumer fears. McDonald's took the leap first, announcing in September 2002 it will switch cooking oils to reduce the amount of trans fatty acids in its food by almost half. Frito-Lay followed suit, unveiling plans to eliminate trans fats from Doritos, Tostitos and Cheetos in the near future.

A Fish Story

Fish, a great source of polyunsaturated omega-3 fats, has received much attention in the past for its potential to lower heart disease risk. And there have been some studies to back this up; however, not all results have consistently showed a benefit. One recent, large trial, however, found that getting 1 gram a day of omega-3 fatty acids (the equivalent of eating 1 serving a day of fatty fish such as mackerel, salmon, sardines and swordfish) over a 3.5 year period could lower the risk of death from heart disease by 25 percent in patients who had a previous heart attack.

Although more research is needed, adding fish to the diet may help lower heart disease risk. The American Heart Association currently recommends that everyone eat at least two servings of fish a week. But it is possible to get too much of a good thing. According to a study conducted by San Francisco internist Jane Hightower, M.D., appearing in the November 2002 issue of the *Journal Environmental Health Perspectives*, 89 percent of Californians who eat fish for lunch and dinner have elevated mercury levels. Obviously, eating fish twice a day on a regular basis is far more than the two servings a week recommendation.

High levels of mercury damage the nervous system, especially in children and fetuses, which is why the Food and Drug Administration recommends that young children and pregnant women limit their fish intake to two 6-ounce cans of tuna each week if that is all the fish they eat, or one can of tuna if they eat other fish. In addition, they should avoid eating swordfish, shark, king mackerel, and tilefish. So how much mercury-tainted fish can cause health problems? That is the question scientists are still struggling to answer.

Fish isn't the only source of omega-3 fatty acids. Other good sources include flax seeds, walnuts, and omega-3 enriched eggs, as well as canola, olive, and flaxseed oils.

Fat and Cancer

Heart disease is not the only condition that is been linked with eating fat. Certain cancers are, too. As with heart disease, it is the type of fat that seems to be important in the relationship, not the total amount of fat.

Breast cancer. The belief that dietary fat was a major cause of breast cancer was very strong by the early 1980s, largely due to international comparisons among countries relating cancer and per capita fat consumption. Such comparisons are very broad in nature, however, and as more detailed studies were performed over the next couple of decades, the link between total fat intake and breast cancer began to evaporate.

Colon cancer. Similar to breast cancer, initial international comparisons associated total dietary fat consumption and the risk of colon cancer. However, later studies contradicted these earlier findings and showed only a weak association. Although the percentage of calories from total fat does not seem related to risk, a high consumption of red meat has been associated with increased risk.

Prostate cancer. Although the exact link between dietary fat and prostate cancer is far from clear, there is some evidence that diets high in animal fat and saturated fat increase the risk of prostate cancer. However, some studies have also shown no association, while others have implicated unsaturated fats. Clearly much more research is needed to clear up the exact link between dietary fat and prostate cancer.

Other cancers. Preliminary research has also linked the intake of certain kinds fat with other cancers, though much more research is needed to confirm these results. In the female nurses study, Harvard researchers found that a high intake of trans fats increased the risk of non-Hodgkin's lymphoma and that a high saturated fat intake increased the risk of endometrial cancer.

Dietary Fat and Obesity

It is a common belief that the more fat you eat, the more body fat you will put on, and the more weight you will gain. This belief has been bolstered by much of the nutritional advice given to people over the past decade, which has focused on lowering total fat intake while increasing carbohydrate intake. Current data show, however, that this advice has been misguided. While total fat intake nationwide has dropped over the last decade, rates of obesity have increased steeply.

Most studies show that over the short term, a low-fat diet does result in weight loss. But many diets show such benefits over the short term. However, there seemed to be no substantial benefit of a low-fat diet compared to a diet with a fat intake close to the national average.

Although more research is needed, a prudent recommendation for losing weight or maintaining a healthy weight is to be mindful of the amount of food you eat in relation to the amount of calories you burn in a day. Exercising regularly is especially beneficial.

Recommendations for Eating Fat

The basic message for eating fat is simple: limit the bad fats and replace them with good ones. Here are a few guidelines:

- Cut down or cut out trans fats.
- Limit saturated fats.
- Add more polyunsaturated and monounsaturated fats.
- You can lower your blood cholesterol level and your risk of heart disease by exercising regularly.

Here are some tips for lowering your trans-fat intake:

- Choose liquid vegetable oils or a soft tub margarine that is contains little or no trans fats.
- Reduce intake of commercially prepared baked goods, snack foods, and processed foods, including fast foods.
- When foods containing hydrogenated or partially hydrogenated oils can't be avoided, choose products that list the hydrogenated oils near the end of the ingredient list.

A common mistake is adding good fats without eliminating bad ones, and maybe also cutting back on some easily digested carbohydrates. Fats pack a lot of calories in a small package (9 calories per gram compared with 4 calories per gram for carbohydrates). So if you aren't careful, adding good fats without cutting back elsewhere in your diet can lead to weight gain, which could offset some of the benefits from eating better fats.

Our Real Needs For Carbohydrates

What are carbohydrates? Carbohydrates are a necessary part of a healthy diet because they provide the body with the energy it needs for physical activity and to keep organs functioning properly. Carbohydrates include sugars, starches and fibers. Many foods rich in whole-grain carbohydrates are also good sources of necessary vitamins and minerals.

The word *carbohydrate* comes from the combination of carbon and water. The simplest carbohydrate is glucose. Glucose, or "blood sugar" and "dextrose," flows in the bloodstream so every cell in your body can absorb it. Your cells absorb glucose and convert it into energy to drive the cell. Specifically, a set of chemical reactions on glucose creates ATP (adenosine triphosphate), and a phosphate bond in ATP powers most of the machinery in any human cell.

Because glucose is the essential energy source for your body, your body has many different mechanisms to ensure that the right level of glucose is flowing in the bloodstream. For example, your body stores glucose in your liver (as glycogen) and can also convert protein to glucose if necessary. Carbohydrates provide the energy that cells need to survive.

Research shows us that carbohydrates' effect on health is fairly complex and greatly depends on not only the amount, but also the type of carbohydrates we eat. Some carbohydrates help promote health, while others may actually increase the risk of diseases like diabetes and coronary heart disease. Carbohydrates are in a wide variety of foods, including beans, milk, popcorn, bread, potatoes, cookies, spaghetti and cherry pie, but there is a difference between the type of carbohydrates found in these foods. As with dietary fat (covered in the next section), there are no hard and fast rules about carbohydrates. Simply, "good" carbohydrates—found in bread, pasta and other starches—have been classified as complex carbohydrates, and simple carbohydrates or sugars—such as table sugar, candy and honey—were considered "bad." Research now shows us, however, that the picture is more complicated than this.

During digestion, all carbohydrates are broken down in the intestine into their simplest form, sugar, which then enters the blood. As blood sugar rises, the body's normal response is to increase levels of the hormone insulin in the blood. Insulin is released by the pancreas to help the body's cells use the blood sugar for energy. This, in turn, helps bring blood sugar levels down to normal levels.

In some people this response does not work properly. For example, people with type II diabetes may not have enough insulin or their insulin may not work well enough to lower the blood sugar. The result may be high blood sugar levels or a condition known as insulin resistance, where both the blood sugar and insulin levels in the blood remain high.

A number of factors promote insulin resistance, including genetics and family history, leading a sedentary lifestyle, being overweight, and eating a diet filled with foods that cause big spikes in blood sugar.

Carbohydrates and the Glycemic Index

Recently, a new type of classification of carbohydrates has evolved, questioning many of the old assumptions of how carbohydrates are related to health. Called the glycemic index, this new classification is a measure of how quickly and how strongly blood sugar rises after eating foods that contain carbohydrates. Diets filled with high glycemic index foods—which can cause quick and strong increases in blood sugar levels—have been linked to an increased risk of both diabetes and heart disease.

A number of factors determine the glycemic index of food. One of the most important is how much the "manufacturer" has processed the carbohydrates are that are in the food. Highly processed carbohydrates—those where the outer bran and inner germ layer are removed from the original kernel of grain—cause bigger spikes in blood sugar levels than less processed grains. Whole-grain foods tend to have a lower glycemic index than their more-processed counterparts. For example, white rice, which is highly processed, has a higher glycemic index than brown rice, which receives less processing.

A number other factors also impact how quickly the carbohydrates in food raise blood sugar levels, including the following:

- **Fiber content.** Fiber helps shield carbohydrates from immediate digestion, so the sugars in fiber-rich foods tend to be absorbed more slowly into the blood stream.
- **Ripeness.** A ripe fruit or vegetable has a higher sugar content than one that is still green and, therefore, has a higher glycemic index.
- **Type of starch.** The type of starch granules in a food influences how fast the carbohydrates are digested and absorbed into the blood stream. The starch in potatoes, for example, is digested and absorbed into the blood stream relatively quickly.
- **Fat content and acid content.** The higher the fat content or acid content of a food, the slower its carbohydrates are converted to sugar and absorbed into the blood stream.
- **Physical form.** Finely ground flour has a higher glycemic index than more coarsely ground flour.

Some foods that contain complex carbohydrates—such as potatoes—quickly raise blood sugar levels, while some foods that contain simple carbohydrates—such as whole fruit—raise blood sugar levels more slowly.

Although the glycemic index seems complex, it's actually quite simple; substitute refined grains, cereals, and sugars with minimally processed whole-grain products whenever possible. And potatoes—

Foods and the Glycemic Index

High Glycemic	Low Glycemic
potatoes	most legumes
french fries	whole fruits
white bread	whole wheat, oats, bran
white rice	brown rice
bananas	bulgur
breakfast cereals	whole-grain breakfast cereals
white spaghetti	whole-wheat pasta
soft drinks	couscous
sugar	barley

once on the complex carbohydrate preferred list—should be eaten only occasionally because of their high glycemic index.

Dieters Beware

A number of popular diets emphasize carbohydrates. Some stress a high level of carbohydrates, while others emphasize a low intake. Examples of high-carbohydrate/very low-fat diets include:

- Dean Ornish
- Pritikin
- Food for Life

For many years, we've all heard the advice to cut back on the total amount of fat we eat and to consume more complex carbohydrates. And thousands of food items in supermarkets come in low-fat alternatives. But research shows cutting back on fat and loading up on carbohydrates is *not* a healthy way to eat and lose weight. Just as we now know not all types of fat are bad, we are learning that not all types of carbohydrate are good either.

It's easy to fall into the "low-fat trap." Fat, gram for gram, has more than twice as many calories as protein or carbohydrates; it seems logical that choosing low-fat products would help with weight loss. However, many of the low-fat products are loaded with sugar to make up for the loss of the "fat taste" many of us crave. So while people think they are hastening weight loss by choosing low-fat alternatives, they could be choosing foods that have just as many, if not more, calories than the full-fat version.

Many people also tend to think because a food is low in fat, they can eat as much of it as they want, and they won't gain weight. As far as the body is concerned though, one calorie is the same as another, no matter where it came from. Eat too many calories—whether they come from fat, carbohydrates, or protein—and you'll gain weight.

The popularity of low-fat food has bigger implications for health beyond losing weight. Many people are increasing the amount of carbohydrates in their diets, particularly in the form of sugars (as we've learned from the glycemic index). Too much sugar can increase the risk of heart disease and diabetes.

For example, in the Harvard Nurses study, researchers calculated that substituting an equal number of calories of polyunsaturated fat with carbohydrates increased the risk of heart disease by over 50 percent. Other studies have also found a low-fat, high-carbohydrate diet (particularly those high-in sugars) can worsen blood cholesterol and triglycerides levels, both of which are risk factors for coronary heart disease.

Low-fat diets are no longer universally thought of as the weight-loss solution they once were. The latest research shows a more prudent approach to fat and carbohydrates in the diet is to not focus on total fat intake but, rather, to substitute the "bad" fats—saturated and trans fats—with "good" fats—polyunsaturated and monounsaturated fats—and to eat more whole grains high in dietary fiber. For weight loss, the best approach is to be mindful of the amount of food you are eating in relation to the amount of calories you are burning in a day. Naturally, an important way to lose weight, or maintain a healthy weight, is regular exercise.

Then there are also low-carbohydrate, high-protein diets. Examples of this type diet programs include:

• The Zone
• Atkins diet
• Gerald Reavan
• Protein Power Lifeplan

In response to the potentially negative effects of high-carbohy-drate, low-fat diets, many diets push in the opposite direction, pro-moting potential benefits of a low-carbohydrate, high-protein diet. Milk, steak, ham, and bacon—the type foods people typically avoid when trying to lose weight—are often featured in these diets. Many of the high-protein foods people choose on these diets are high in saturated fat and low in vitamins and minerals. Saturated fat can increase the risk of heart disease and colon cancer. Diets very high in protein—especially animal protein, like red meat—can also increase the risk of osteoporosis in women because the body takes calcium from the bone to neutralize the acids in the blood that builds up from the digestion of large amounts of protein.

Although gaining in popularity, initial results from studies show that people might lose weight over the short term on a high-pro-tein diet, but this may simply be due to the fact that those on the high-protein diet were eating fewer calories, something that often happens when people drastically change how they eat. Whether a high-protein diet results in sustained, long-term weight loss needs further study.

Recommendations for Eating Carbohydrates

Until more is known about the true risks and benefits of these low-carbohydrate, high-protein diets, they should be viewed with caution. Research shows protein consumption should be kept at moderate amounts—about 8 grams of protein a day per 20 pounds of body weight—and focus largely on vegetable protein. Focus on carbohydrate-rich foods—in the form of whole grains, fruits, and vegetables.

Our Real Needs for Fiber

Fiber is one of those things that many of us know is important, but we're not real sure what it is and what its health benefits are. Fiber is present in all plants that are eaten for food, such as fruits, vegetables, grains, and legumes.

Not all fiber is the same, however, and there are a number of ways to categorize it. One is by where the fiber came from. For

example, fiber from grains is referred to as cereal fiber. Another is
to categorize it by how easily it dissolves in water. Soluble fiber partially dissolves in water. Insoluble fiber does not dissolve in water.
These differences are important when it comes to fiber's effect on
the risk of disease.

Sources of Fiber

Soluble Fiber
- oatmeal
- nuts and seeds
- dried peas
- lentils
- pears
- blueberries

- oat bran
- legumes
- beans
- apples
- strawberries

Insoluble Fiber
- whole grains
- couscous
- bulgur
- whole-grain breakfast cereals
- seeds
- cucumbers
- celery

- barley
- brown rice
- whole-wheat breads
- wheat bran
- carrots
- zucchini
- tomatoes

Current recommendations suggest that adults consume 20 to 35
grams of dietary fiber per day. Children over the age of two years
should consume an amount equal to or greater than their age plus
5 grams per day. On a daily average, Americans eat only 14 to 15
grams of dietary fiber.

Health Effects of Eating Fiber

Long heralded as part of a healthy diet, fiber appears to reduce
the risk of conditions such as heart disease, diabetes, diverticular
disease, and constipation. As I said in a previous chapter, despite
what many people may think, fiber probably has little, if any, effect
on the risk of colon cancer.

Here's a summary of the effect of fiber on other chronic diseases:

Heart disease. Coronary heart disease is a leading cause of death for both men and women in the U.S. It is characterized by a build up of cholesterol in the coronary arteries (the arteries that feed the heart), which causes them to become hard and narrow, a process referred to as atherosclerosis. A total blockage of a coronary artery results in a heart attack. A high dietary fiber intake has been linked to a lower risk of heart disease in a number of large studies that followed people for many years. Cereal fiber, the fiber found in grains, seems especially beneficial.

Type II diabetes. This is the most common form of diabetes and is characterized by sustained high blood sugar levels. It tends to develop when the body is no longer able to produce enough of the hormone insulin to lower blood sugar to normal levels, or to properly use the insulin that it does produce. There are several important factors that may help lower risk of type II diabetes, such as maintaining a healthy weight, being physically active, and not smoking. Researchers are also trying to pinpoint dietary factors that may lower the risk of type II diabetes, one of which seems to be a high-fiber diet. Studies of both the male health professionals and female nurses have found that a diet high in cereal fiber was linked to a lower risk of type II diabetes.

When it comes to factors that increase the risk of diabetes, a diet low in cereal fiber and at the same time high in high-glycemic index foods, foods that cause big spikes in blood sugar, seems particularly bad. Both the study of nurses and health professionals found that this diet combination more than doubled the risk of type II diabetes compared to a diet high in cereal fiber and low in high-glycemic index foods.

Foods that have a high-glycemic index include potatoes, refined foods such as white bread, white rice, refined cereals (corn flakes, Cheerios), white spaghetti and sugar. Foods with a low-glycemic index do not raise the blood sugar as fast and, therefore, are associated with a lower risk of type II diabetes. Low glycemic index foods include legumes, whole fruits, oats, bran and whole-grain cereals.

Diverticular disease. Fiber has long been used in the prevention of diverticulitis, an inflammation of the intestine that is one of the most common disorders of the colon among the elderly in Western societies. In North America, this painful disease is estimated to occur in one-third of all persons over forty-five years of age and in two-thirds of all persons over age eighty-five. The Harvard study of male health professionals found that eating dietary fiber, specifically insoluble fiber, was associated with about a 40 percent lower risk of diverticular disease.

Constipation. This is the most common gastrointestinal complaint in the United States and is particularly of concern to the elderly. The gastrointestinal tract is highly sensitive to dietary fiber, and consumption of fiber seems to relieve and prevent constipation. The fiber in wheat bran and oat bran seem to be more effective than similar amounts of fiber from fruits and vegetables. Experts recommend increasing fiber intake gradually rather than suddenly. The intake of water and other noncaffeinated beverages should also be increased, as fiber absorbs water. Healthy people should drink at least eight 8-ounce glasses of water each day.

Recommendations for Eating Fiber

Fiber is an important part of a healthy diet, and you should get at least the minimum recommended amount of 20 to 35 grams of dietary fiber per day for adults. For children over two years old, the recommended intake is age plus 5 grams. The best sources of fiber are fresh fruits and vegetables, nuts and legumes and whole-grain foods.

Here are some tips that will help improve your fiber intake:

• Eat whole fruits instead of drinking fruit juices.
• Substitute white rice, bread and pasta with brown and whole-wheat versions.
• Incorporate whole-grain cereals for breakfast.
• Snack on raw vegetables instead of chips, crackers or chocolate bars.
• Substitute legumes for meat two to three times per week in chili and soups.
• Experiment with international dishes—such as Indian or middle-eastern—featuring whole grains and legumes as part of the main meal or as part of salads.

Our Real Needs for Water

Our bodies are one-half to four-fifths water, depending on how much body fat a person has. Water makes up more than 75 percent of our brains, about 80 percent of our blood and about 70 percent of our lean muscle.

Since water is vital to not just our health, but also to our survival, we've all heard the advice: drink plenty of water. Yet surveys indicate that many Americans don't drink enough.

Every system in our bodies depend on water, which performs the following functions:

* regulates your body temperature
* removes wastes
* carries nutrients and oxygen to your cells
* cushions your joints
* helps prevent constipation
* lessens the burden on your kidneys and liver by helping flush some of the toxins
* helps dissolve vitamins, minerals and other nutrients to make them accessible to your body

Lack of water can lead to dehydration. Even mild dehydration of as little as 1–2 percent loss of your body weight can sap your energy and make you lethargic. Dehydration poses a particular health risk for the very young and very old.

Disease Prevention

Besides helping our bodies run smoothly, some evidence shows that water helps prevent certain diseases.

Kidney stones. People who have had kidney stones often can prevent further stones from forming by drinking lots of fluid.

Colon cancer. One study found that women who drank more than five glasses of water a day had a risk of colon cancer that was 45 percent less than those who drank two or fewer glasses a day.

Bladder cancer. There's also some evidence that water consumption can help prevent bladder cancer. A study of more than forty-seven thousand men who took in an average of more than 2.5 quarts of fluid each day, including water, were found to have a lower risk of bladder cancer than men who drank less than half as much.

Heart disease. Drink five or more 8-ounce glasses of water a day and a lot less of almost every other kind of liquid, and you'll significantly lower your risk of coronary heart disease. Researchers at Loma Linda University in California conducted a "lifestyle survey" in 1976 with people thirty-eight years and older who were living in California Seventh-Day Adventist households. They received responses from 8,280 men and 12,017 women. The participants were followed for six years, and during that time 246 respondents died from heart disease. Dr. Jacqueline Chan, the lead researcher, concluded that women who drank more than five 8-ounce glasses of water each day were 41 percent less likely to die from a heart attack during the study period than those who drank two or fewer glasses daily. For men who drank a lot of water, the heart attack risk dropped by 54 percent.

The opposite also is noteworthy. Women who drank less water and more coffee, tea, juice, and milk had a twofold increased risk of death. For men, it carried a 46 percent increase of a heart attack death. Why? What's so magic about water? Chan says water is absorbed in the blood, decreasing the blood's "thickness." This in turn lowers the risk of developing a heart attack-triggering blood clot. When our bodies digest fluids other than water, the digestive process pulls water out of the blood to dilute whatever it is we have consumed.

What Do the "Experts" Say?

On average, most adults lose about 10 cups (2.4 liters) of fluid a day through sweating, exhaling, urinating and bowel movements. Logic dictates that you need to take in 10 cups of water each day to compensate. As you'll soon see, not everyone agrees.

Although water often is your best choice, drinking water isn't the only way to replace those fluids. For instance, you can get water from other beverages and from food. Just how much water you need to drink each day depends on what you eat, your sex, how active you are, the weather, your health, your age and the medications you may be taking. Exercising or engaging in any activity that causes you to perspire and dehydrate increases your water requirement, as do hot, humid or cold weather and high altitudes. The National Research Council (NRC) uses a sliding scale of 1 milliliter of water for every calorie burned. This scale is not for women who are pregnant or breastfeeding, infants, children and older adults who are unhealthy. The NRC says the average man who burns about 2,900 calories daily needs 2,900 milliliters, or about 12 cups, of water each day. The average woman who burns 2,200 calories daily needs about 2,200 milliliters, or about 9 cups, of water each day. For your own calculations: One measuring cup of water equals 236 milliliters of water.

Solid food also contains water. In an average diet, food provides about 3 to 4 cups of water each day. Men, because they generally are bigger and have more lean muscle tissue, need more water on average than women do each day.

You can also meet part of your water requirement by drinking fluids such as milk, juice and soup, but watch your intake of caffeinated beverages, soda and alcohol. Caffeine is mildly dehydrating and large amounts of caffeine cause jitters, irritability, insomnia and elevated blood pressure. Alcohol, besides being dehydrating, is addicting, can impair physical performance and mental functioning, and is associated with increased risk of some diseases. Soda contains sugars and other calories that can inhibit weight loss and cause tooth decay.

The amount of water you drink needs to increase if you are active or outside in hot or humid weather. To determine whether you're getting enough water in your day, look at the color of your urine. If your urine is pale yellow, you're probably drinking enough fluids. If your urine is dark yellow and has a strong odor, or if you go to the bathroom less than four times a day, you probably need to increase your water intake.

If you're healthy and not in any dehydrating conditions, some experts say that you can use your thirst as an indicator of when to drink. Others believe that if you're thirsty, you've already started to dehydrate. Thirst is not always an adequate indicator of your body's need for fluid replenishment during exercise. Studies show that during vigorous exercise an important amount of your fluid reserves may be lost before you're aware of thirst. Make sure you are sufficiently hydrated before, during and after exercise. Also, the older you are, the less you're able to sense that you're thirsty, so drink up.

Increased thirst and increased urination (both in volume and frequency) can be symptoms of diabetes. With diabetes, excess blood sugar (glucose) in your body draws water from your tissues, making you feel dehydrated. To quench your thirst, you drink a lot of water and other beverages, and that leads to more frequent urination. If you notice unexplained increases in your thirst and urination, see your doctor. It may not necessarily mean you have diabetes. It could be something else. And some people consume excessive amounts of water and experience increased urine output not associated with any underlying disease.

When it comes to water, play it safe. Make a conscious effort to keep yourself hydrated. Drink a glass of water with each meal and between each meal. Keep a bottle with you during the day or take regular water breaks. Getting enough water just might buoy your health.

A Dissenting Opinion

It has become accepted wisdom to drink at least eight glasses of water a day. Everywhere you go, people carry bottles of water, constantly sipping from them. It's becoming acceptable to drink water anywhere, anytime. In fact, a pamphlet distributed at one southern California university even tells its students to "carry a water bottle with you. Drink often while sitting in class . . ."

A Dartmouth Medical School physician thinks the advice is unnecessary. Heinz Valtin, M.D., says the universal advice that has made guzzling water a national pastime is more urban myth than medical dogma and appears to lack scientific proof. In a review published online by the *American Journal of Physiology* August 8, 2002, Valtin, professor emeritus of physiology at Dartmouth Medical School, reports no supporting evidence to back this popular counsel, commonly known as "eight by eight" (referring to drinking 8 eight-ounce glasses of water daily).

Valtin, a kidney specialist and author of two widely used textbooks on the kidney and water balance, sought to find the origin of this dictum and to examine the scientific evidence, if any, that might support it. He observes that we see the exhortation everywhere: from health writers, nutritionists, even physicians. Valtin doubts its validity. Indeed, he finds it, "difficult to believe that evolution left us with a chronic water deficit that needs to be compensated by forcing a high fluid intake."

Valtin thinks the notion may have started when the Food and Nutrition Board of the National Research Council recommended approximately "one milliliter of water for each calorie of food," which would amount to roughly two to two-and-a-half quarts per day (64–80 ounces). Although in its next sentence, the Board stated "most of this quantity is contained in prepared foods," that last sentence may have been missed, so the recommendation was erroneously interpreted as how much water one should drink each day.

He found no scientific studies in support of eight glasses a day recommendation. Rather, surveys of fluid intake on healthy adults of both genders, published as peer-reviewed documents, strongly suggest that such large amounts are not needed. His conclusion is supported by published studies showing that caffeinated drinks, such as most coffee, tea and soft drinks, may indeed be counted toward the daily total. He also points to the quantity of published experiments that attest to the capability of the human body to maintain proper water balance.

Valtin emphasizes that his conclusion is limited to healthy adults in a temperate climate leading a largely sedentary existence—precisely, he points out, the population and conditions that the "at least" in the "eight by eight" refers to. At the same time, he stresses that large intakes of fluid, equal to and greater than 8 eight-ounce glasses, are advisable for the treatment or prevention of some diseases, such as kidney stones, as well as under special circumstances, such as strenuous physical activity, long airplane flights or hot weather. But barring those exceptions, he concludes that we are currently drinking enough and possibly even more than enough.

Despite the dearth of compelling evidence, then, what's the harm? "The fact is that, potentially, there is harm even in water," explains Valtin. Even modest increases in fluid intake can result in "water intoxication" if one's kidneys are unable to excrete enough water (urine). Such instances are not unheard of, and they have led to mental confusion and even death in athletes, in teenagers after ingesting the recreational drug Ecstasy, and in ordinary patients.

He lists other disadvantages of a high water intake: (a) possible exposure to pollutants, especially if sustained over many years; (b) frequent urination, which can be both inconvenient and embarrassing; (c) expense, for those who satisfy the "eight by eight" requirements with bottled water; and (d) feelings of guilt for not achieving the eight-glass standard.

Other claims discredited by scientific evidence that Valtin discusses include the following:

Thirst is too late. It is often stated that by the time people are thirsty, they are already dehydrated. On the contrary, thirst begins when the concentration of blood (an accurate indicator of our state of hydration) has risen by less than two percent, whereas most experts would define dehydration as beginning when that concentration has risen by at least five percent.

Dark urine means dehydration. At normal urinary volume and color, the concentration of the blood is within the normal range and nowhere near the values that are seen in meaningful dehydration. Therefore, the warning that dark urine reflects dehydration is alarmist and false in most instances.

Is there scientific documentation that we do not need to drink "eight by eight"? There is highly suggestive evidence, says Valtin. First is the voluminous scientific literature on the efficacy of the osmoregulatory system that maintains water balance through the antidiuretic hormone and thirst. Second, published surveys document that the mean daily fluid intake of thousands of presumably healthy humans is less than the roughly two quarts prescribed by the eight-glasses-a-day standard. Valtin argues that, in view of this evidence, the burden of proof that everyone needs 8 eight-ounce glasses should fall on those who persist in advocating the high fluid intake without, apparently, citing any scientific support.

Finally, strong evidence now indicates that not all of the prescribed fluid need be in the form of water. Careful peer-reviewed experiments have shown that caffeinated drinks should indeed count toward the daily fluid intake in the vast majority of persons. To a lesser extent, the same probably can be said for dilute alcoholic beverages, such as beer, if taken in moderation.

"Thus, I have found no scientific proof that absolutely every person must 'drink at least eight glasses of water a day,'" says Valtin. While there is some evidence that the risk of certain diseases can be lowered by high water intake, the quantities needed for this beneficial effect may be less than 8 eight-ounce glasses, and the recommendation can be limited to those particularly susceptible to the diseases in question.

Not So Fast . . .

A Ball State University professor disagrees with Valatin's recommendations and subsequent news stories claiming drinking eight glasses of water per day might not be important for all people. Katherine Beals, nutrition professor, contends that reporters may have misinterpreted the interview in the *Journal of Applied Physiology*. She says after the journal article was made public, several news reports may have misinterpreted it to mean the 64-ounce standard was unnecessary for everyone, she said. "However, it is not applicable to most people, particularly athletes and active individuals who probably need more than 64 ounces of fluid per day."

The average sedentary person loses about 2 to 2.5 liters daily while athletes and active people can lose far more, said Beals, a triathlete. "The old standard of consuming eight glasses containing eight ounces of water is a good one for anyone, especially for active individuals" she said. "You will need more fluid to replace the fluid loss if you lead an active lifestyle, which includes physical activities, physical labor and living or working in a warm place."

Recent news stories also picked up on the journal article's claim that people don't have to drink water, but can find fluid from other foods, such as fruits, vegetables and cereals.

"You can certainly get fluids from other sources, such as fruits and vegetables," Beals said. "However, the average American typically consumes two servings or less of fruits and vegetables daily. Most people eat meats and breads, which contain little fluid. If we depended on food for our fluids, we'd all be dehydrated."

Beals also disagreed with reports that caffeinated beverages do not lead to dehydration. Because caffeinated drinks have a diuretic effect, they are not as effective at maintaining hydration as noncaffeinated beverages and should not be the sole source of fluid consumed in a day.

There's no doubt our bodies need water, and if you choose to lug around a bottle all day, it's doubtful you'll cause yourself any harm. Finding the right water balance for each of us is important and depends on our body size, level of physical activity, exercise and sweating, the local climate, and our diet. Once you find that level there's one other critical point; the water you're drinking must be pure and free of contaminants.

Cool, Clear Water?

We are making huge demands on our fresh water supplies by our lifestyle, while at the same time introducing complicated mixtures of chemicals into the water that we drink. Being totally mobile water can carry contamination from place to place with the greatest of ease.

Prior to the late 1960s the availability of clean drinking water was not considered to be a problem. Although stories in the media hinted at troubles on the horizon, knowledgeable scientists studying the extent of the pollution of water supplies, began realizing the full extent of the coming water contamination problems.

Chlorination is used extensively by municipal water treatment plants to disinfect water. Chlorine is used almost universally in the treatment of public drinking water because of its toxic effect on harmful bacteria and other water-borne, disease causing organisms. But there is a growing body of scientific evidence that shows chlorine in drinking water may actually pose greater long-term dangers than those for which it was used to eliminate. These effects of chlorine may result from either ingestion or absorption through your skin.

What concerns health officials are the chlorination by-products, "chlorinated hydrocarbons," known as trihalomethanes (THMs). Most THMs are formed in drinking water when chlorine reacts with naturally occurring substances such as decomposing plant and animal materials.

Scientific studies have linked chlorine and chlorination by-products to cancer of the bladder, liver, stomach, rectum and colon, as well as heart disease, atherosclerosis (hardening of the arteries), anemia, high blood pressure and allergic reactions. There is also evidence that shows that chlorine can destroy protein in the body and cause adverse effects on skin and hair. The presence of chlorine in water may also contribute to the formation of chloramines in the water, which can cause taste and odor problems. Since chlorine is required by public health regulation to be present in all public drinking water supplies, it is up to you to remove it at the point of use in your home.

Three out of four Americans are concerned about the safety of their tap water, which has led to a dramatic increase in sales of water filtration systems and bottled water. About five billion gallons of bottled water were guzzled in the United States in 2000.

Good, clean water is not a given. Most city waters, and even wells, are suspect for contamination with microbes and chemicals.

Water Purification

You should consider buying a water filtration system. The best is a reverse osmosis unit or a solid carbon block type filter; what's most effective for your home use depends on what your water concerns are and how much water you need. Many people also buy bottled water from natural springs or water bottled after filtration.

Bottled water is regulated by the Food and Drug Administration. Even so, a four-year test of bottled brands by the environmental resource group Natural Resources Defense Council found that one-third of the brands contained bacteria or other chemicals that exceeded industry guidelines. Most of the water tested, however, was fine.

If you prefer bottled to tap water, read the label carefully to be sure that you're not paying top dollar for "spring water" that's actually bottled from a municipal water supply.

One more caveat. If you drink water from a bottle, refill or replace the bottle often. Every time you drink, the bacteria from your mouth contaminate the water in the bottle. To keep it clean, wash your container in hot, soapy water or run it through a dishwasher before refilling it.

The Food and Drug Administration (FDA) regulates bottled water, and in 1996, new standards went into effect. So bottled water quality is improving, but it's still good to shop around for the best. Here are descriptions of a variety of bottled waters that will be good to know while shopping around:

Artesian water. Drawn from a confined aquifer (rock formation containing water) in which the water level stands above the natural water table.

Distilled water. Evaporated and then condensed, leaving it free of dissolved minerals.

Purified water. Demineralized water, produced by deionization (passing it through resins that remove most of the minerals) or by reverse osmosis (passing it through filters to remove dissolved solids). Distilled water also is considered purified water.

Mineral water. Contains no less than 250 parts per million (ppm) of total dissolved, naturally occurring (not added) solids, or minerals. Mineral water can be labeled low mineral content (less than 500 ppm) or high mineral content (more than 1,500 ppm).

Spring water. Obtained from an underground formation from which water flows naturally to the surface, or it may be collected through a bore drilled into the spring.

Sparkling water. Containing carbon dioxide gas either naturally ("natural sparkling water") or synthetically—this gas has been added to it.

Seltzer water. Also sparkling water. The name comes from the town of Niederselters in the Weisbaden region of Germany. Seltzer was introduced in the late 1700s and is considered the forerunner of soda pop.

Soda water. A carbonated water that contains sodium bicarbonate.

Club soda. Same as soda water except that mineral salts such as bicarbonate, citrate and phosphate have been added.

Tonic water. Carbonated and flavored with fruit extracts, sugar and quinine (a bitter alkaloid).

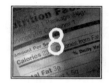

Our Real Needs for Micronutrients

The vitamins and minerals we consume are known as micronutrients. We need micronutrients for normal growth, body function and health. Your body can't make most micronutrients, so you must get them from either the foods you eat or the supplements you take. Typically, foods are better since they provide multiple nutrients and other important compounds.

The function of nutrients is a complex process, occurring every second within our cells. In school, you might have learned how each nutrient functioned individually, as well as the role each played in helping other nutrients to function. A marginal nutrient deficiency could interrupt the biochemical balance, and a prolonged deficiency could result in more serious clinical conditions.

Vitamins, or the lack thereof, impact normal body functions, mental alertness and resistance to infection. They enable our bodies to process proteins, carbohydrates and fats. Certain vitamins also help produce blood cells, hormones, genetic material and nervous system chemicals. If these micronutrients are missing during phases of rapid growth, the development of basic biological functions like intellect, and even life itself, can be threatened. This is why young children and pregnant women are often among the risk groups for micronutrient deficiencies.

Vitamins and minerals don't supply calories for fuel. That is the job of the macronutrients: carbohydrates, proteins and fats. Micronutrients do, however, help our bodies release and use calories gained from macronutrients.

There are fourteen recognized vitamins, usually categorized as "fat-soluble" or "water-soluble." For your information, I've marked those vitamins and minerals that are antioxidants with an asterisk (*).

Fat-soluble vitamins, which are stored in body fat, inlcude:

- vitamin A*
- vitamin D
- vitamin E*
- vitamin K

If too much vitamin A and vitamin D are consumed, they can reach toxic levels. (More on that later.)

Water-soluble vitamins, which are stored in the body to a lesser extent than fat-soluble vitamins, include:

- vitamin C *
- choline
- biotin
- thiamin (B1)
- riboflavin (B2)
- niacin (B3)
- pantothenic acid (B5)
- pyridoxine (B6)
- folic acid/folate (B9)
- cobalamin (B12)

Major minerals (those needed in larger amounts), include:

- calcium
- phosphorus
- magnesium
- sodium
- potassium
- chloride

Table 8.1 100% Daily Value of Vitamins

VITAMIN	100% Daily Value (current RDI)
Vitamin A	5000 IU
Vitamin C	60 mg
Vitamin D	10 mcg
Vitamin E	20/30 mg*
Vitamin K	80 mcg
Thiamin	1.5 mg
Riboflavin	1.7 mg
Niacin	20 mg
Pantothenic acid	10 mg
Vitamin B6	2 mg
Folic acid	400 mcg
Vitamin B12	6 mcg
Biotin	300 mcg

* The first figure refers to the vitamin E obtained from a natural source while the second figure refers to synthetically created vitamin E.

Table 8.2 100% Daily Value of Minerals

MINERAL	100% Daily Value (current RDI)
Calcium	1000 mg
Chloride	3400 mg
Chromium	120 mcg
Copper	2 mg
Iodine	150 mcg
Iron	18 mg
Magnesium	400 mg
Manganese	2 mg
Molybdenum	75 mcg
Phosphorus	1000 mg
Potassium	3500 mcg
Selenium	70 mcg
Zinc	15 mg

Calcium, phosphorus and magnesium are important to the development and health of bones and teeth. Sodium, potassium and chloride, known as electrolytes, are important in regulating the water and chemical balance in our bodies.

In addition, the body needs smaller amounts of these minerals:

• chromium
• copper
• fluoride
• iodine
• iron
• manganese
• molybdenum
• selenium *
• zinc *

Warning! Toxicity

It's vital to our health that we have the right balance of vitamins and minerals in our bodies. Too much of some vitamins and minerals can cause toxic reactions as you can see from table 8.3.

Even though most nutrients are safe, some can be dangerous and too much of anything can be toxic. The fat-soluble vitamins that can accumulate in the body, such as vitamins A and D, are of particular concern. Acute toxicity usually results from one or two large doses, and chronic toxicity usually refers to months of supplementation or excessive exposure to high amounts in water or food. The nutrient with the greatest risk of toxicity is vitamin A, especially for children and pregnant women.

Many minerals themselves are toxic in large doses. For some, the body insists on a critical balance among them to function effectively. If this balance is disrupted by a megadose of one mineral, a relative shortage of another may be the result. For example, too much phosphorus increases the need for calcium and may produce a calcium deficiency, even if you're consuming calcium in recommended amounts.

Other minerals, such as iron and magnesium, can be stored in the body and may build up to produce toxic symptoms. And most of the so-called trace minerals, which are needed in only tiny

Table 8.3 Potenially Toxic Dosages and Side Effects of Nutrients

Nutrient	Toxic Dose	Symptoms and Diseases
Biotin	n/a	No side effects from oral administration at therapetic doses reported
Boron	10 mg	No side effects reported
Calcium	2,000 mg	Drowsiness, extreme lethargy, impaired absorption of iron, zinc and manganese, calcium deposits in tissues throughout body, mimicking cancer on x-ray
Carotene	300 mg	Orange discoloration of skin, weakness, low blood pressure, weight loss, low white cell count
Chromium	50 mg	Dermatitis, intestinal ulcers, kidney and liver impairment
Copper	15 mg	Fatigue, poor memory, depression, insomnia, increased production of free radicals, may suppress immune function. Violent vomiting and diarrhea. Cooking acid foods in unlined copper pots can lead to toxic accumulation of copper.
Fluoride, acute	500 mg	Poisons several enzymes (5,000 mg can be lethal)
Fluoride, chronic	5 mg	Fluorosis (white patches on teeth), bone abnormalities
Folic Acid	15 mg	Abdominal distention, loss of appetite, nausea, sleep disturbance, interferes with zinc absorption, may prevent recognition of vitamin B12 deficiency
Iodine	2 mg	Thyroid impairment, iodine poisoning or sensitivity reaction
Iron	25 mg	Intestinal upset, interferes with zinc and copper absorption, loss of appetite, not safe for those with

Table 8.3 continued

Nutrient	Toxic Dose	Symptoms and Diseases
Magnesium	n/a	iron storage disorders such as hemosiderosis, idiopathic hemo-chromatosis, or thalassemias. Toxic build-up in liver, pancreas, and heart. Diarrhea at large dosages of poorly absorbed forms (like Epsom salts). Disturbed nervous system function due to calcium-to-magnesium ratio imbalance; catharsis, hazard to persons with poor kidney function.
Manganese	75 mg	Toxicity only reported in those working in manganese mines or drinking from contaminated water supplies, which results in loss of appetite, neurological damage, loss of memory, hallucinations, hyperirritability, elevation of blood pressure, liver damage, mask-like facial expression, blurred speech, involuntary laughing, spastic gait, hand tremors.
Niacin, acute	50 mg	Transient flushing, headache, cramps, nausea, vomiting
Niacin, chronic	3 g	Anorexia, abnormal glucose tolerance, gastric ulceration, elevated liver enzymes. Excessive uric acid in blood, possibly leading to gout.
Pantothenic acid	n/a	Occasional diarrhea. Increased need for thiamin, possibly causing thiamin deficiency symptoms.
Phosphorus	n/a	Distortion of calcium-to-phosphrus ratio, creating relative deficiency of calcium.
Potassium	n/a	Mental impairment, weakness. High potassium in blood, causing paralysis and abnormal heart rhythms.

Table 8.3 continued

Nutrient	Toxic Dose	Symptoms and Diseases
Vitamin B6	300 mg	Sensory and motor impairment. Dependency on high doses, leading to deficiency symptoms when one returns to normal amounts.
Riboflavin	n/a	No toxic effects have been noted. See Thiamin.
Selenium	750 mcg	Diabetes, garlic-breath odor, immune impairment, loss of hair and nails, irritability, pallor, skin lesions, tooth decay, nausea, weakness, yellowish skin
Thiamin	n/a	No toxic effects noted for humans after oral administration. However, since B vitamins are interdependent, excess of one may produce deficiency of others.
Vitamin A, acute (infant)	75,000 IU	Anorexia, bulging fontanelles, hyper-irritability, vomiting
Vitamin A, acute (adult)	2,000,000 IU	Headache, drowsiness, nausea, vomiting
Vitamin A, chronic (infant)	10,000 IU	Premature epiphyseal bone closing, long bone growth retardation
Vitamin A, chronic (adult)	50,000 IU	Anorexia, headache, bluffed vision, loss of hair, bleeding lips, cracking and peeling skin, muscular stiffness and pain, severe liver enlargement and damage, anemia, fetal abnormalities (pregnant women must be very careful), menstrual irregularities, extreme fatigue, liver damage, injury to nervous system.
Vitamin B12	n/a	No side effects from oral administration have been reported. (See thiamin)
Vitamin C, acute	10 g	Nausea, diarrhea, flatulence
Vitamin C, chronic	3 g	Increased urinary oxalate and uric acid levels in rare cases, impaired carotene utilization, chelation (bind-

Table 8.3 continued

Nutrient	Toxic Dose	Symptoms and Diseases
Vitamin C, chronic		ing of vitamin C with minerals) and resultant loss of minerals may occur, sudden discontinuation can cause rebound scurvy. Kidney and bladder stones, urinary tract irritation, increased tendency for blood to clot, breakdown of red blood cells in persons with certain common genetic disorders (such as glucose-6-phosphate dehydrogenase deficiency, common in persons of African origin)
Vitamin D, acute	70,000 IU	Loss of appetite, nausea, vomiting, diarrhea, headache, excessive urination, excessive thirst
Vitamin D, chronic	10,000 IU	Weight loss, pallor, constipation, fever, hypercalcaemia. In infants, calcium deposits in kidneys and excessive calcium in blood; in adults, calcium deposits throughout the body (may be mistaken for cancer) (pregnant women must be careful), deafness, nausea, kidney stones, fragile bones, high blood pressure, high blood cholesterol, increased lead absorption.
Vitamin E	1,000 IU	The safe dose is probably over 2,000 IU, but some people experience weakness, fatigue, exacerbation of hypertension, increased activity of anticoagulants at 1,000 IU, although some research shows that as little as 300 IU can slow down the immune system. Can destroy some vitamin K made in the gut. A small amount of immune

Table 8.3 continued

Nutrient	Toxic Dose	Symptoms and Diseases
Vitamin E		suppression is probably a reasonable trade off for vitamin E's much needed antioxidant activity.
Vitamin K	n/a	No known toxicity with natural (phylloquinone); synthetic (menadione), although relatively safe, when administered to infants may cause hemolytic and liver enlargement. Anemia in laboratory animals.
Zinc	75 mg	Gastrointestinal irritation, vomiting, adverse changes in HDL/LDL cholesterol ratios, impaired immunity. Nausea, anemia, bleeding in stomach, premature birth and stillbirth, abdominal pain, fever. Can aggravate marginal copper deficiency. May produce atherosclerosis.

SOURCES: USDA and National Academy of Science

quantities, are deadly poisons in doses much beyond the amounts essential for good nutritional health.

Warning! Deficiencies

Although vitamin deficiencies such as scurvy or beriberi aren't much of a problem in the U.S. today, other prolonged vitamin or mineral deficiencies can cause specific diseases or conditions such as the following:

• night blindness (vitamin A deficiency)
• pernicious anemia (vitamin B12 deficiency)
• anemia (iron deficiency)

If some of these micronutrients are lacking in the diet there are recognizable symptoms. For example, lack of iodine can cause an enlarged thyroid gland, known as goiter, recognizable by the unsightly swelling on the throat. Other deficiencies may cause more general signs such as weakness, paleness and lack of resistance to infections.

The three major micronutrient deficiencies emphasized by the World Health Organization (WHO) worldwide are:

* vitamin A
* iron
* iodine

Vitamin A Deficiency

Vitamin A has been focused on not only because of the blindness it can cause, but because it is essential to the body's maintenance of many functions, especially the immune system, which protects against infection. It's believed many children in developing countries would have been saved from dying from different infections, particularly measles, if they had adequate and available vitamin A in their diet.

Fortunately, this deficiency is easy to correct. Foods chock full of vitamin A are plentiful in red, yellow and orange fruit and vegetables; in dark, green, leafy vegetables; and in most animal products like milk, meat, and especially liver.

Iron Deficiency

Iron is a fundamental mineral for the making of hemoglobin (a substance carrying oxygen in to the tissues of the body) in the red blood cells. It usually results from having a diet low in easily absorbable iron, which is often aggravated by increased iron demands due to pregnancy, child and pubescent growth spurts and losses through menstruation or intestinal worms.

If this deficiency is not treated, it eventually leads to low hemoglobin, a condition known as anemia, which may result in symptoms and signs ranging from weakness, tiredness, reduced learning ability to increased risk of infection, and even death during childbirth.

Iodine Deficiency

Iodine is a chemical element used by the thyroid gland to produce hormones that regulate the bodily metabolism. In the U.S., much of our table salt is fortified with iodine. The consequences of this deficiency include goiter (an unsightly swelling of the thyroid gland in front of the neck), reduced mental function and increased risk of stillbirths, abortions and infant deaths. Iodine-deficient women may give birth to babies with severe mental and neurological impairment. If this deficiency occurs during infancy or childhood, it causes irreversible mental retardation, growth failure, speech and hearing defects, among others. Even mild deficiency may cause a low intellectual capacity.

Unlike vitamin A and iron, this deficiency is very difficult to deal with by education and better eating habits, because either iodine is present in the environment where foods are produced, or it is not.

Our best defense against nutrient deficiency is eating micronutrient rich foods such as (in the case of vitamin A deficiency) yellow and orange fruits and dark green leafy vegetables. Many of us don't bother with these foods because we don't like them, or we don't realize their importance. Sometimes one nutrient can boost your absorption of another. In the case of iron deficiency, iron absorption from food is increased by eating foods rich in vitamin C such as citrus fruits among many others.

By no means are these the only deficiencies and sometimes the effectiveness of one nutrient is dependent on others. For example, vitamin D is required to help the bones absorb calcium or calcium supplements. (For a complete list of deficiencies, see chart 8.4.)

Drug Interference

Some drugs can contribute to nutrient deficiencies. Drugs and food can interact in various ways. Some drugs can decrease or increase nutrient absorption, and others can change the processes by which the body uses nutrients or eliminates excess foods. Medications can also affect appetite or taste perception, changing food intake. For example, medications prescribed for inflammatory bowel disease (IBD) have long been associated with nutritional deficiencies. Inadequate food intake, inflammation of the small

Table 8.4 Vitamin Deficiencies

Nutrient	Toxic Dose	Symptoms and Diseases
Niacin	14–19 mg/day	Skin inflammation (especially upon exposure to sunlight) diarrhea, edema. *Note sustained release products have a higher incidence (rate) toxicity—avoid unless recommended by your physician
Riboflavin	1–1.4 mg/day	Bleeding gums. inflammation of mucous membrane of the mouth and/or nose
Thiamin	0.8–1.1 mg/day	Fatigue, depression, irritability, fast heart rate, swelling in extremities, lowered body temperature, disorientation, pins and needle sensation in hands and feet
Vitamin A	2600–3300 IU	Dry, scaly skin, "corkscrew" hair, night blindness, dryness of eye sockets
Vitamin B6	1.1–1.8 mg/day	Nausea, vomiting, sores on mucous membranes (especially inside mouth) pins and needles sensation in hands and feet
Vitamin B12	1 mcg/day	No known symtoms of deficiency.
Vitamin C	30–40 mg/day	Scurvy, seen as spongy, bleeding gums, loose teeth, loss of appetite, weakness, joint pain
Vitamin D	100 IU/day	Bone tenderness and fragility, rickets
Vitamin E	9–13 IU/day	Edema, skin lesions, breakdown of blood cells (rare in adults)

Source: CDS, FDA, USDA, National Academy of Science

intestine, and diarrhea are often responsible for these deficiencies. However, many of the drugs used to treat IBD can also contribute to nutritional difficulties.

Here are the effects of common drugs prescribed to treat IBD according to the Crohn's & Colitis Foundation of America, Inc.

Sulfasalazine

Sulfasalazine not only inhibits the absorption of folic acid, but also interferes with its breakdown into a form the body can use. Thus, the use of sulfasalazine in IBD patients can cause a folic acid deficiency. Symptoms include sore mouth, diarrhea, irritability, and forgetfulness. If the deficiency progresses, it can lead to anemia. To prevent this, people taking sulfasalazine are encouraged to eat foods rich in folic acid, such as liver, lean beef, veal, yeasts, leafy vegetables, legumes, fruits, eggs, potatoes and whole grain cereals. Yet, patients also must be careful with raw fruits and vegetables, which might aggravate symptoms. If you cannot receive an adequate amount of folic acid through dietary measures, supplements can be prescribed. The usual dose is 1 mg daily.

Corticosteroids

Corticosteroids may cause the body to eliminate potassium at a greater rate, leading to a deficiency in some patients. Thus, you may need to increase the potassium in your diet. Some food sources are whole and skim milk, bananas, prunes and raisins. If patients taking long-term corticosteroids develop a potassium deficiency, doctors can prescribe a supplement.

Corticosteroids also may suppress calcium absorption, in addition to directly decreasing bone formation. Thus, patients who take these drugs have an increased risk of developing a calcium deficiency. Long-term corticosteroid use increases this risk, which in turn raises the risk of osteoporosis. Calcium deficiency is a key concern in children with IBD, since it could lead to a stunting or retardation of growth.

To prevent corticosteroid-induced calcium deficiency and adverse effects on bone, patients need to increase their calcium intake. Increased consumption of dairy products, however, could be a problem if you are lactose intolerant. Commercially available lactase enzyme supplements may help you digest milk products. If you cannot tolerate these foods, nonprescription calcium supplements, such as calcium carbonate, are recommended. Vitamin D supplements may be prescribed for persons at high risk for developing bone problems. Multivitamins with added calcium generally do not contain enough to serve as the only daily calcium substitute.

Other Medications

Other, less commonly used drugs can cause nutritional problems. For example, methotrexate is associated with decreases in folic acid absorption, and cyclosporine can aggravate a magnesium deficiency. Consult your doctor about your diet if you are taking these drugs. In short, people with IBD should be aware that drugs can cause or aggravate nutritional disorders. Fortunately, your diet can be modified or supplemented to meet additional needs and help prevent complications.

Whole Foods

Whole foods usually provide a synergy between the micronutrients the food contains. This is why it can be dangerous to supplement with only one nutrient. For example, you can get your entire RDA of vitamin C (which as it stands is too low) by taking a pill, or by eating a large orange. The orange, a whole food, is much, much better because it provides fiber, beta-carotene and other valuable nutrients along with the vitamin C.

Whole foods—fruits, vegetables, grains, lean meats and dairy products—have three main benefits you can't find in a pill:

- *Whole foods are complex.* They contain a variety of the nutrients your body needs—not just one. For example, the orange provides not just vitamin C but also beta-carotene, bioflavonoids, calcium and other nutrients. A straight vitamin C supplement lacks these other nutrients.
- *Whole foods provide dietary fiber.* Fiber is important for healthy

digestion and to help prevent certain diseases. Soluble fiber (found in certain beans and grains and in some fruits and vegetables) and insoluble fiber (found in whole grains and in some vegetables and fruits) may help prevent heart disease, diabetes and constipation.

• *Whole foods contain other substances that may be important for good health.* Fruits and vegetables, for example, contain naturally occurring food substances called phytochemicals, which may help protect you against cancer, heart disease, osteoporosis and diabetes. Although it's not yet known precisely what role phytochemicals play in nutrition, research shows many health benefits from eating more fruits, vegetables and grains. If you depend on supplements rather than eating a variety of whole foods, you miss the potential benefits of phytochemicals. I'll tell you more about phytochemicals shortly, as well as other key substances we need.

Only well-designed, long-term studies can sort out which nutrients in food are beneficial and whether taking them in pill form provides the same benefit. In fact, some nutrients may actually be harmful to your health when taken as a supplement. In one study, researchers found an increased risk of prostate cancer among men who drank alcohol and took beta-carotene supplements. In an earlier study, they found that smokers who took beta-carotene supplements had an increased risk of lung cancer. It's possible that alcohol and tobacco change the way your body absorbs and uses beta-carotene. In addition, large amounts of beta-carotene can alter blood levels of other, similar natural food pigments called carotenoids, some of which may actually be more beneficial to you than beta-carotene.

We should concentrate on getting our nutrients from food, though, not supplements. Whole foods provide an ideal mix of nutrients, fiber and other food substances. It's likely that all of these work in combination to keep you healthy.

In the case of Mother Nature versus science, science takes a back seat. There's no doubt Mother Nature knows much, much more about nutrients than supplement "designers."

What Do "Fortified" and "Enriched" Mean?

We often see the words *fortified* or *enriched* on food and beverage packaging. These terms indicate that nutrients have been added. If a food or beverage is fortified, it means that one or more nutrients have been added that weren't originally there.

Enriched means that the nutrients lost during processing have been added back. The Nutrition Facts listed on the label will tell you which nutrients have been added. It'll also show what percent of the Daily Value for each nutrient is met with one serving.

These terms aren't necessarily a good thing. Often, perfectly fine and vital nutrients are squeezed out during processing and others, sometimes replicas, of the originals are added back later. Again, Mother Nature is much wiser than those in the food science laboratory. One important exception is folic acid added to cereals and other foods, as you'll see in a later chapter.

It's important to note, food colorings, preservatives and other chemicals ARE NOT enriching or fortifying.

Nutritional Enemies

We're learning more and more that certain diseases could likely be the result of nutrient deficiencies. Even if we're trying to eat right much of our food contains what some call "anti-nutrients." As I've said before and you probably already know, much of today's diet consists of over-processed food—often nutrient depleted and loaded with chemicals that not only do anything good for us but can cause real harm.

An anti-nutrient is any food or component with no real food value in itself. Foods that are so over-refined as to be barely recognizable from its original form also fit this category. There are also "bad," oxygen-derived byproducts from these anti-nutrients called "free radicals," which are dangerous oxidizing substances.

Frankly, our bodies aren't designed to consume free radicals, and they struggle to adapt. Unless kept in check, free radicals can wreak havoc in our bodies. Nutrient deficient bodies simply do not have the quantity of enzymes and antioxidants required to neutralize the effect of free radicals. So these very damaging substances are either left in to run free in our systems until they're excreted or are stored in the only place our body can put them: our cells, fat, and muscle tissue.

Some of the worst anti-nutrient substances include:

- alcohol
- caffeine
- chlorine
- emulsifiers
- fluoride
- food colorings
- flavor enhancers
- herbicides
- nicotine
- pesticides
- prescription and over-the counter drugs
- preservatives
- synthetic hormones
- trans-fatty acids in margarine and unsaturated vegetable oils
- soft drinks
- white, refined sugar and flour

All of these substances increase our need for high-quality nutrients, which assist us to stay healthy, while our body fights the invaders. When our bodies become overwhelmed by anti-nutrients our bodies become weakened and prone to illness and disease. Coupled with all the things that can tax our bodies, for example, people working under stress burn off greater quantities of all B-group vitamins, anti-nutrient buildup can result in organ/system failure, premature aging and eventually disease.

Nutrient deficiency and toxic overload have been linked to many acute and chronic medical conditions such as insomnia, poor concentration, memory loss, blood clots, depression, chronic fatigue syndrome, irritability, yeast infections, hyperactivity, scaly skin, acne, obesity and gum disease. Toxic overload can cause or contribute to migraine headaches, asthma, diabetes, heart disease, hypertension, rheumatoid arthritis and cancer. It can also play a huge part in contracting colds, the flu and other infectious conditions.

What About Supplements?

It is common knowledge that many people either don't eat enough or do not eat balanced meals. Then there are people with medical conditions, pregnant women, the elderly and others who may have increased needs for specific nutrients. This increased need is one reason why so many people turn to supplements.

An FDA survey shows that about 40 percent of the general population take supplements daily, with women taking more than men. Among the elderly, surveys show that between 66 and 72 percent take supplements.

It's also estimated that 5 to 10 percent of the people who take supplements ingest megadoses (defined by some researchers as ten times the USRDA or more) of certain vitamins and minerals.

If you're wondering whether your personal vitamin program is safe, it's not always easy to find out. Although the RDAs/DRIs offer guidelines for everyone, despite what the government says, we're not all alike. "There are no reference guides or tables you can check to see what levels of vitamins trigger harmful effects," points out Paul Saltman, Ph.D., a professor of biology doing research in nutrition at the University of California at San Diego. "That's because the danger levels vary from person to person and depend on factors such as weight, health status, metabolism, diet, nutritional status, the form of the nutrient and how often you take it.

Choosing and Using Supplements

- *Supplements are not substitutes.* They can't replace the hundreds of nutrients in whole foods you need for a nutritionally balanced diet. However, if you do decide to take a vitamin or mineral supplement, here are important points to remember:
- *Look for the USP logo on the label.* This ensures that the supplement meets the standards for strength, purity, disintegration and dissolution established by the testing organization, U.S. Pharmacopeia (USP).
- *Look for expiration dates.* Supplements can lose potency over time, especially in hot and humid climates. If a supplement doesn't have an expiration date, don't buy it.

- *Store all vitamin and mineral supplements out of the sight and reach of children.* Put them in a locked cabinet or other secured location. Don't leave them sitting out on the counter and don't rely on child-resistant packaging. Be especially careful with any supplements containing iron. Iron overdose is a leading cause of poisoning deaths among children.
- *Store supplements in a dry, cool place.* Avoid hot, humid storage locations, such as the bathroom.
- *Explore your options.* If you have difficulty swallowing, ask your doctor whether a chewable or liquid form of the vitamin and mineral supplements might be right for you.
- *Check with your doctor.* Before taking anything other than a standard multivitamin-mineral supplement of 100 percent DV or less, check with your doctor, pharmacist or a registered dietitian. This is especially important if you have a health problem or are taking medication. High doses of niacin, for example, can result in liver problems. In addition, supplements may interfere with your medications. Vitamins E and K, for example, aren't recommended if you're taking blood-thinning medications (anticoagulants) because they can complicate the proper control of blood thinning. If you're already taking an individual vitamin or mineral supplement and haven't told your doctor, discuss it at your next checkup.
- *Never go over dosages above the toxicity level* without the expert guidance of a physician skilled in nutritional medicine.

On this last point, while some people can take more of a nutrient than the toxic dosage and experience no ill effects, some can experience a toxic effect at even lower dosages. You should be able to tell if you're having a negative reaction to a supplement. Even at lower dosages, always monitor yourself carefully and respect the feedback your body provides.

Here's an example. Jane Brody, the *New York Times* columnist and author of *Jane Brody's Nutrition Book* recently reported the following case:

> A forty-six-year-old actress had suffered for three years from weird, debilitating symptoms, including muscular weakness, weight loss, and severe abdominal pain. Her career was destroyed and she could barely walk before doctors realized

Want to Know What's in Your Food?

In August 2002, the Agricultural Research Service launched an updated version of its database that reports all the nutrients in 6,220 food items. Named the "Nutrient Database for Standard Reference, Release 15" (SR15 for short), it is the most complete source of food composition in the U.S. From cheese crackers to chicken patties, salsa to salmon, chances are you'll find it in SR15. Both generic and brand-name food items are included.

Information is derived from U.S. Department of Agriculture research, qualified food industry sources, USDA-sponsored contracts and rigorously evaluated scientific literature.

A single food item's complete profile boasts 117 nutrient categories, appearing in columnar format. Newly developed algorithms are used to evaluate data for scientific accuracy, and quality-control programs maximize data reliability.

Meat product categories in particular have been beefed up. Ground beef data were revamped to reflect new market trends and the demand for low-fat products. Nutritive profiles were added for a variety of emu, ostrich, deer, bison and elk products as well as for eight new beef cuts. Many brand-name, ready-to-eat breakfast cereals and candies were updated to reflect current names and nutrient values.

she was suffering from lead poisoning as a result of taking bone meal, prescribed by her doctor for menstrual cramps. Her self-designed effort to preserve her health by taking megadoses of calcium and other minerals in the form of bone meal had backfired completely. She hadn't known—and none of the twenty-two doctors she saw thought to ask—that bone meal could be hazardous. However, since bones help to protect the body from toxic substances like lead by removing them from the blood and storing them, bone meal can be a source of dangerous substances.

Expensive Urine?

Whenever we take anything into our bodies, our systems metabolize it. The body will use what it can and discard the rest. People who take supplements often notice a change in the color of their urine and rightfully conclude it's caused by nutrients being excreted (usually riboflavin). But if it's being flushed many conclude by swallowing supplements their purchasing nothing more than expensive urine. They're wrong.

It's commonly accepted that most adult Americans do not eat enough fruits and vegetables on a daily basis. The truth is, researchers are finding some nutrients can provide benefits beyond simply preventing nutritional deficiencies. For example, few argue against the potential benefits of vitamin E as it applies to cardiovascular health. Nearly 75 percent of neural tube defects may be prevented by taking increased amounts of folic acid before and during the first trimester.

As Dr. Walter Willet of Harvard University told *Newsweek* in June 1993, "Until quite recently, it was taught that everyone in the country gets enough vitamins through their diet and that taking vitamin supplements just creates expensive urine. I think we have proof this isn't true."

Expensive urine? No more than much of the food, prescription drugs or anything else we put inside our body. Whatever the body metabolizes and uses is beneficial including vitamins. Your body will use and metabolize them and break down the rest to be eliminated. But even that can be an advantage. On its "way out," excess vitamin C protects the bowel, kidneys and bladder on the way out.

So if you consume too much of certain vitamins are you producing expensive urine? Probably, but if no more expensive than eating a costly gourmet meal and certainly much less than bowel surgery. Expensive urine? Maybe, but worth every "scent."

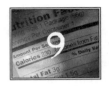

Our Real Needs
for Antioxidants

Here's one of Mother Nature's biggest paradoxes: the same oxygen we breathe and need to live, is also a grave threat to our health. Here's how. As our bodies perform their normal metabolic processes, some of the oxygen molecules we inhale lose an electron. When this happens, the formerly stable oxygen molecules become dangerous free radicals. In excess, free radicals travel through the body producing harmful oxidation that cause damage to cells and genes by snagging electrons from other molecules. This process is called oxidation.

Over time, free radicals can increase our risk of nearly two hundred diseases including cardiovascular disease, cancer, cataracts, arthritis and can even damage our DNA. For one thing, scientists believe free radicals speed up hardening of the arteries by causing cholesterol to oxidize before it develops or settles within the artery walls. (Many believe antioxidants might help prevent this process.) Free radicals can also contribute to premature aging since, as we age, our ability to repair these attacks is reduced.

Still, free radicals play an important role in our bodies, and a certain amount are absolutely necessary for life. Free radicals promote beneficial oxidation by helping convert air and food into chemical energy at the cellular level. Free radicals are also a crucial part of the immune system, attacking foreign invaders including bacteria. It's the excess amounts that cause trouble.

The production of free radicals and the destruction of excessive amounts in a benign manner is the result of normal metabolic processes. Ideally, antioxidants mop the damaging ones up. Simply put, antioxidants grab hold of these free radicals, "grabbing" them so that they cannot cause any more damage. They then bind the free radical to another chemical that also prevents it from causing damage on a more permanent basis, and the antioxidant goes back to find another free radical. In a perfect world, this system works just fine. But since we don't live in a perfect world, problems occur.

Antioxidants, which include certain vitamins and minerals and a variety of other substances, are available to us in the foods we eat—especially fruits and vegetables—and as supplements. It is known that people who eat adequate amounts of antioxidant-rich foods have a lower incidence of health problems including cardiovascular disease, certain cancers and cataracts.

Antioxidants can do many things for us, including:

- reduce cholesterol
- slow down the aging process
- reduce the risk from many types of cancers
- help the body fight carcinogens
- suppress tumor growth
- reduce risk of arteriosclerosis
- help protect against heart disease and stroke
- slow down progression of Alzheimer's disease
- protect eyes from macular degeneration, the most prevalent cause of vision loss in people over sixty-five
- defend the body against ravages from cigarette smoke
- protect the body from chronic obstructive pulmonary disease (COPD) such as asthma, bronchitis, and emphysema
- counteract environmental pollution

Good Stuff, Wouldn't You Say?

The greatest danger to our health today is chronic degenerative disease. Heart disease, cancer and strokes are our chief killers, while arthritis, chronic fatigue and a host of other debilitating conditions are destroying the quality of life of millions of people. Research now shows moderate to high levels of antioxidants can alleviate many of these deadly and distressing diseases including reducing the risk of cancers of the lung, uterus, cervix, mouth and gastrointestinal tract. Plus, antioxidants might very well slow aging and reduce degenerative disease.

For instance, it's believed Parkinson's and Alzheimer's disease can be caused in part by oxidative stress. Recent research shows antioxidants can help prevent Alzheimer's disease and slow the progress of Parkinson's disease.

Here's more good news. Antioxidants can protect against cataracts and reduce the risk of macular degeneration by 43 percent. Also, antioxidants can reduced asthma, and they can help children with cystic fibrosis. Plus, antioxidants protect against emphysema and alleviate arthritis.

Unfortunately, the modern, typical diet—especially inadequate amounts of fruits and vegetables—plus environmental factors, keeps us from consuming enough antioxidants to fight off free radicals. As a result, antioxidants are overtaxed trying to scavenge free radicals generated by any the following:

- cigarette smoke, including second-hand smoke
- pollution
- chemicals
- drugs
- alcohol
- excessive consumption of processed foods
- grains grown in leached soil
- fatty foods
- cured meats
- foods containing chemicals such as preservatives, additives, colorings and pesticide residues

The soil for growing crops today are depleted of minerals after decades of over use and the application of nitrogen, phosphorus and potassium fertilizers. As a result, most of us have deficiencies in magnesium, selenium, zinc and chromium in our diets increasing our risk of degenerative disease.

But even if we're conscientious, and manage to take in the nutrients we need, we breathe in car fumes and fumes from resins, paints, aerosols and indoor chlorinated pools. We absorb chemicals through the skin from skin care products, shampoos and conditioners, make-up and sunscreens. Some of these chemicals are toxic—even carcinogenic. An estimated five hundred thousand new man-made chemicals have been released since World War II. This means half a million new chemicals are impacting our bodies that our ancestors were never exposed to. In the body they contribute to excessive amounts of free radicals.

Although the theory of free radical and oxidative stress was first advanced in 1956, we are still in our infancy stage in understanding all we need to know about antioxidants. What we do know is each is different; they work in different places, at different times, and in different dosage.

There have been a few reports in the media suggesting high levels of antioxidant vitamins and minerals are a health hazard. The truth is, the only risk of taking moderate to high levels of antioxidants are that high levels of vitamin C can be laxative, vitamin E can thin the blood and selenium may cause hair loss and brittle nails. Doses of 400–1,200 IU vitamin E per day has been shown to inhibit platelet adhesion. The use of vitamin E to thin the blood in the prevention and treatment of heart disease is surely preferable to using warfarin, a rat poison, commonly prescribed for this purpose.

There are no recorded cases of people killing themselves with a vitamin overdose that I know of. Compare that to the tens of thousands of people dying every year from medicines at the prescribed dose. *The Journal of the American Medical Association* reports that it's not unusual for prescribed drugs to kill over a one hundred thousand people in a year with more than two million hospitalized. Granted, many of the people taking prescription drugs are trying to ward off a terminal illness and for some the death is only postponed. Still, drug reactions are now the fourth major cause of death after heart disease, cancer and stroke. Visiting a doctor is more likely to put your health at risk than visiting a health food store. This is not meant as an indictment of the health care system and workers. No one can deny the value of modern medicine in emergencies, and we know drugs do save lives. But, research shows antioxidants can also save lives but without the risk of serious side effects.

Women and Antioxidants

Are antioxidants more important for women than men? It is too soon to say, but one study suggests women experience more oxidative stress from cell-damaging free radicals than men.

In the study, a research team led by Dr. Gladys Block of the University of California at Berkeley measured oxidative damage in 298 healthy adults who ranged in age from nineteen to seventy-eight. The study included 138 cigarette smokers, 92 nonsmokers and 68 people who reported exposure to secondhand smoke.

The researchers measured levels of two substances: malondialdehyde and F2-isoprostanes—both known markers of oxidative damage. These byproducts are produced after fatty substances called lipids are oxidized.

Based on levels of these markers, oxidative damage was significantly more extensive in women than in men. In fact, female sex was a more powerful predictor of oxidative damage than smoking.

The higher level of oxidative damage in women was unexpected, and the researchers do not have a good explanation for it. At first, Block and her colleagues thought that the higher percentage of body fat in women might be to blame, but when they accounted for body mass index (BMI)—a measurement that considers both weight and height—women still had higher levels of oxidation.

The finding of higher levels of oxidative stress in women is particularly important, say the authors, since "women have been found to be at greater risk of lung cancer than men exposed to similar levels of cigarette smoke."

The researchers report that people with higher levels of a substance called C-reactive protein—a marker of inflammation that has been linked to heart disease—also tended to have more oxidative stress. By contrast, oxidative stress was lower in people who ate the most fruit as well as in those who had higher blood levels of vitamin C and carotenoids—pigments in fruits and vegetables that the body uses to make vitamin A.

However, neither smoking, age, alcohol use nor other dietary factors affected levels of oxidative stress. Likewise, a form of vitamin E called alpha-tocopherol did not seem to influence oxidative stress, the report indicates. The study appeared in the *American Journal of Epidemiology* in mid-2002.

The RDA/DRI Antioxidant List

Antioxidants included in the government's RDA/DRI nutritional standards include:

• vitamin A
• vitamin C
• vitamin E
• selenium
• zinc

This is a pretty slim list considering how many antioxidant compounds there are, including well-known substances such as beta-carotene, which the body converts into vitamin A. The government seems determined to only include vitamins and minerals. What about the other substances, such as caretonoids, flavonoids, and isoflavones? Well, they aren't considered nutrients and don't make their list even though they're packed into a wide variety of fruits, vegetables and grains. I'll talk about them in the next chapter.

Below I've listed the government's guidelines for each of the antioxidant vitamins and minerals. These are for reference only. As I've said before, and I think it bears repeating, the "one-size-fits-all" guidelines don't take into consideration our own personal situations. For example, it is very difficult to calculate or even measure our state of health because it is in constant fluctuation. We can measure health according to a number of parameters: exposure to viruses and bacteria, exposure to allergens, physical and emotional stresses, and dietary abuse—such as too much sugar, caffeine, alcohol and tobacco. Also, our emotional and psychological sense of well-being affects many of the body's metabolic processes.

As a starting point for antioxidants, let's start with those on the RDA/DRI list.

Vitamin A

The maximum daily intake (from all sources) unlikely to pose a risk of side effects for adults is 10,000 IU per day. Some experts recommend a maximum of 5,000 IU per day for pregnant women.

Vitamin A is a fat-soluble vitamin and is part of a group of compounds called retinoids. Vitamin A plays an important role in vision, bone growth, reproduction, cell division and cell differentiation, the process by which a cell decides what it is going to become. Vitamin A also may help prevent bacteria and viruses from entering your body by maintaining the integrity of skin and mucous membranes. It also maintains the surface linings of our eyes and respiratory, urinary and intestinal tracts. When those linings break down, bacteria can enter our bodies and cause infection.

Vitamin A also helps our bodies regulate its immune system. The immune system helps prevent or fight off infections by making white blood cells that destroy harmful bacteria and viruses. Vitamin A helps lymphocytes, a type of white blood cell that fights infections, function more effectively. Inadequate amounts of vitamin A can cause vision impairment, especially at night.

Our bodies convert plant sources of beta-carotene into vitamin A, but animal sources of vitamin A are better absorbed. So, vegetarians who rely on fruits and vegetables rich in beta-carotene to meet their daily vitamin A requirement need to eat at least five daily servings of such foods. Actually, we all do, but few of us bother.

Two national surveys in the 1990s indicated that some Americans don't eat enough foods rich in vitamin A. Although vitamin A deficiency is rare in the United States (it's more often associated with malnutrition, a leading problem in developing countries), we're not taking advantage of its disease-preventing ability.

For people with certain diseases who have trouble absorbing vitamin A, doctors often recommend supplements. However, studies show diets rich in vitamin A and beta-carotene from food (not supplements) provide the added protection against some types of cancer.

Table 9.1 RDA and DRI for Vitamin A

Life Stage	Men	Women	Pregnant	Breastfeeding
Age 19+	3,000 IU	2,330 IU	–	–
Other	–	–	2,565 IU	4,335 IU

Table 9.2 Vitamin A RDA/DRI for Children

Age	1–3	4–8	9–13	14–18 male	14–18 female
DRI for children	1,000 IU	1,330 IU	2,000 IU	3,000 IU	2,330 IU

Excess alcohol intake depletes vitamin A from your body and is associated with reduced vitamin A intake. It is very important for anyone who consumes excessive amounts of alcohol to include good sources of vitamin A in his or her diet. Vitamin A supplementation may not be recommended for individuals who abuse alcohol because alcohol may increase liver toxicity associated with excess intakes of vitamin A.

Retinol is one of the most active, or usable, forms of vitamin A, and is found in animal foods such as liver and eggs. Retinol is often called preformed vitamin A. Maybe you've heard the term retinoids, which are compounds chemically similar to vitamin A. Over the past fifteen years, synthetic retinoids have been prescribed for acne, psoriasis, and other skin disorders. Isotretinoin is considered an effective anti-acne therapy. At very high doses it can be toxic, which is why this medication is usually saved for the most severe forms of acne.

Too much vitamin A stored in our bodies can increase the risks of birth defects and liver abnormalities and may reduce bone mineral density, resulting in osteoporosis. If you're pregnant or breast-feeding, don't take vitamin A in doses greater than the RDA for pregnant or breast-feeding women.

Food sources. Animal sources include whole milk, whole eggs, liver, beef and chicken. Most fat free milk and dried nonfat milk solids sold in the U.S. are fortified with vitamin A to replace the vitamin A lost when the fat is removed. Fortified foods such as fortified breakfast cereals also provide vitamin A.

Plant sources providing beta-carotene, which converts into vitamin A, include dark green leafy vegetables and orange and yellow fruits, such as carrots, sweet potatoes, spinach, broccoli, cantaloupe, mangos, apricots, butternut squash, turnip greens, bok choy, mustard greens, and romaine lettuce, as well as vegetable soup and tomato juice.

It is best when vitamin A is consumed through the diet rather than through supplements. Also, cooking increases the bioavailability of carotenoids in plant foods, and absorption of vitamin A from the diet is improved when consumed along with some fat in the same meal.

Side effects. Signs and symptoms of vitamin A toxicity include nausea and vomiting, headache, dizziness, blurred vision and problems with muscular coordination. Most cases of vitamin A toxicity result from an excess intake of vitamin A supplements. Plant sources of beta-carotene, which converts to vitamin A, are generally considered safe. A high intake of beta-carotene from plant sources can turn your skin an orange color, but this is not considered a health concern. However, the safety of beta-carotene supplements is questionable.

Vitamin C

Vitamin C, also known as ascorbic acid or ascorbate, is a water-soluble vitamin. Besides it's antioxidant properties, which help prevent cell damage, vitamin C maintains skin integrity, helps heal wounds and is important in immune functions. Humans are one of the few species who lack the enzyme to convert glucose to vitamin C.

Studies show people who eat foods high in vitamin C have lower rates of cancer and heart disease, though it's unclear

Table 9.3 RDA and DRI for Vitamin C

Life Stage	Men	Women	Pregnant	Breastfeeding
Age 19+	90 mg	75 mg	–	–
Adult (smokers)	125 mg	110 mg	–	–
Other	–	–	85 mg	120 mg

whether taking vitamin C supplements produces similar benefits. A 2001 study indicates that supplementation with vitamin C, certain other antioxidants and zinc may slow the progression of age-related macular degeneration, a disease of the eye; but a doctor's supervision is important to determine proper doses to lower the risk of side effects. The Institute of Medicine states that there are no established benefits for consuming vitamin C in doses higher than the RDA. Other research has suggested that 200 mg per day is the optimal dose. Not everyone agrees.

Vitamin C is probably the most controversial substance in nutrient history. Its biggest proponent was the late Linus Pauling, who won Nobel prizes in 1954 for chemistry and in 1962 for peace. Dr. Pauling believed that daily megadoses of vitamin C could prevent cancer—and could also cure cancer.

Pauling wrote three books in support of vitamin C: *Vitamin C and the Common Cold*, *Vitamin C and Cancer* and *How to Live Longer and Feel Better*. In these books he quoted extensive experimental support for his conclusion that vitamin C has a general antiviral effect, which protects against any virus including influenza, polio, hepatitis, mononucleosis and herpes. But its effects are not confined to its ability to defend against viruses and bacteria.

Pauling argues that patients with cancer usually have very low concentrations of vitamin C in the blood plasma and in the blood leucocytes. This lack prevents the leucocytes from doing their job of engulfing and digesting bacteria and other foreign cells, including malignant cells, in the body. He felt that it was reasonable to suppose that the low level of vitamin C indicated it was being used up in the effort to control the disease. By giving patients a larger amount of vitamin C their bodily defenses should therefore be strengthened. Further evidence came from epidemiological studies that showed higher cancer incidence among people whose vegetable and vitamin C intakes were low.

Pauling teamed up with a Scottish doctor, Ewan Cameron. Cameron had come to the same conclusion by another route: malignant tumors produce an enzyme, hyaluronidase, which attacks the intercellular cement of the surrounding healthy tissues. This weakens the cement to such an extent that the cancer is able to invade. Cameron suggested that one way of defending against the cancer might therefore be to strengthen the intercellular cement. Since vitamin C is involved in the synthesis of collagen (the material of which the intercellular cement is composed), high doses of vitamin C should have the effect of strengthening these defenses by allowing faster synthesis. This should protect against the spread and growth of a tumor.

Cameron and Pauling started to experiment with vitamin C on terminal cancer patients at Vale of Leven Hospital in Scotland over the next few years. They carried out a controlled study, comparing the outcome of one hundred patients who were randomly assigned to Dr. Cameron's care to the outcome of one thousand patients assigned to doctors who did not believe in or use vitamin C therapy. They discovered the patients treated with a daily 10 grams of sodium ascorbate had a survival time 4.2 times longer than for patients who did not take such large doses. A significant percent of the terminally ill cancer patients expected to die in weeks or months went on to live much, much longer. In effect, they were cured.

Pauling took these results back to the National Cancer Institute in the U.S. who said they were only interested in animal studies. When Pauling applied for grants to conduct this animal-based research he was turned down eight times. Eventually, he made a point of what was happening by publishing an advertisement seeking private donations to help him continue his research. In a *Wall Street Journal* advertisement he wrote, "Our research shows that the incidence and the severity of cancer depends on diet. We urgently want to refine that research so that it may help to decrease suffering from human cancer. The U.S. Government has absolutely and continually refused to support Dr. Pauling and his colleagues during the past four years."

Eventually pressure built up and the Mayo Clinic was asked to conduct clinical trials of vitamin C. One study, conducted in 1985, by Dr. Moertel at Mayo, and widely reported in the press, showed no evidence that vitamin C had any beneficial effect on cancer patients. In his research, Dr. Moertel conducted a double-blind clinical trial that showed no difference between the survival of those who had been given vitamin C and those who had been given a placebo.

Pauling was very critical of this trial. In 1986, Pauling wrote "[Moertel] suppressed the fact that the vitamin C patients were not receiving vitamin C when they died and had not received any for a long time (median 10.5 months). [This misrepresentation] has done great harm. Cancer patients have informed us that they are stopping their vitamin C because of [these] negative results."

Why was the U.S. National Cancer Institute so quick to support a negative result for vitamin C and so slow to support positive findings? Critics point to the fact that the pharmaceutical industry is well represented in the committees and subcommittees of all of the leading cancer-related institutions. If it were ever found that vitamin C was indeed a powerful anticancer agent, then the pharmaceutical companies would lose an important part of their business. Some scoffed at this notion, arguing doctors wouldn't turn down any substance that had a reasonable chance of curing cancer. Perhaps so; however, today many doctors and researchers take for granted that vitamin C might, in fact, help ward off cancer.

Vitamin C and Lung Disease

In a study reported in the May 2002 *American Journal of Respiratory and Critical Care Medicine*, researchers found people who consume high levels of vitamin C and magnesium tend to have healthier lungs. And for the first time, the research showed that people with high levels of vitamin C intake experience a lower decline in lung function over time.

By minimizing the decline in lung function as time passes, a diet containing lots of foods rich in vitamin C may lower the odds of developing chronic obstructive pulmonary disease (COPD). Mounting evidence suggests that vitamin C and other antioxidant vitamins and minerals may be involved in asthma and COPD, a group of illnesses that includes bronchitis and emphysema. Exactly how antioxidants keep lungs healthy is uncertain, though they are known to neutralize DNA-ravaging compounds called free radicals that contribute to aging and disease.

Previously, Tricia M. McKeever and colleagues at the University of Nottingham in the U.K. found in a study of more than two thousand six hundred adults that high levels of vitamin C and magnesium both corresponded with healthier lungs based on a measure of lung function called forced expiratory volume 1, or FEV1. Nine years later, when the researchers were able to follow up with a little more than half of the original study participants, they confirmed these findings.

"High vitamin C and magnesium intake are associated with higher levels of lung function," said McKeever. "Over a period of nine years, those with higher levels of intake of vitamin C experienced less severe decline in lung function than those with lower levels of intake," she added.

Can Vitamin C Help You Lose Weight?

Losing weight by taking vitamin C is a complicated process, and the researchers aren't positive it works. In other words, more tests are needed. But their theory makes sense. As we get older, when free radicals are formed the resulting oxidative stress on our bodies are greater, resulting in tissue damage and interference with normal physiological functions. University of Colorado at Boulder researchers think oxidative stress may also cause a lowered resting metabolism. In other words, increased oxidative stress in older adults could prevent the nervous system from doing its job and supporting resting metabolism. As a result, fewer calories are burned, resulting in weight gain.

What might be a good way to overcome the oxidative stress? Antioxidants. And the best way to get antioxidants is by eating a diet rich in fruits and vegetables.

To test their theory, the University of Colorado researchers injected vitamin C directly into the veins of study participants, all of whom were sixty to seventy-four years old. Following the vitamin C infusion, resting metabolism increased on average by almost 100 calories a day, which led the research team to theorize that the vitamin C removed oxidative stress.

This has huge implications for reducing age-associated weight gain, as well as reducing the risks for cardiovascular and metabolic diseases such as diabetes.

How Much Vitamin C Should You Take?

The RDA/DRI amounts, although they can ward off scurvy, hardly make a dent in all the potential benefits from much greater amounts of vitamin C. So what's the most you should take? Frankly, there is no maximum level of vitamin C that will cause ill health or toxicity. The complaint that it could lead to kidney stones has never been proven.

It appears that no matter how much we take we can never reach a dose that is toxic. There are two reasons for this. Firstly, the body handles vitamin C in large quantities. Secondly, if the body gets more vitamin C than it can handle at any one time it dumps the excess vitamin C by causing diarrhea, which stops as soon as vitamin C levels become manageable again. This diarrhea-causing amount will vary from person to person. Known as the bowel tolerance level, it will normally be in the region of 10–20 grams a day for a healthy adult but it will increase sharply to 30–60 grams or even more if there is a viral infection. Research shows our bodily reserves of vitamin C fluctuate according to how much is needed to buttress the immune system, scavenge free radicals, regulate cholesterol and sugar metabolism, repair wounds, etc.

Going back to vitamin C pioneer and proponent, Linus Pauling's argument: This increased ability to tolerate higher levels of vitamin C during periods of ill-health suggests that the body is capable of using more vitamin C at times of ill-health. This leads to the conclusion that the body is using the vitamin C to fight the illness. So one measure of the optimum daily amount would be an amount slightly less than the bowel tolerance level.

Let's look at this from another angle. Humans are one of a small group of animals that don't produce vitamin C in their bodies. (We share this defect with the other apes and, curiously, with the guinea pig.) For us, vitamin C has to be taken from food. Most mammals, however, manufacture vitamin C in their livers through the action of a particular enzyme; and they do so in large quantities. A goat for example produces approximately 13 grams a day per 70 kilograms (kg) of body weight under normal conditions, but if it gets stressed it will produce up to 100 grams or more. Mice produce 275 mg of vitamin C per kilo of body weight a day under normal conditions. A mouse the size of a 70 kg man would therefore be producing 19 grams a day. These amounts can increase tenfold when the animal is under stress. Since humans are mammals, we almost certainly need vitamin C in quantities similar to other mammals of the same size and weight. Secondly, if animals produce more vitamin C when they are under stress then presumably, the vitamin C is useful to help the body cope with stress, and illness is a form of physical stress.

Those who believe in the "expensive urine" argument should consider this:

- The urinary system is very prone to infection, so it actually makes sense to direct an antiviral and antibacterial agent like vitamin C through this system. People who don't have "expensive urine" may be more prone to urinary infections.
- The presence of vitamin C in the urine does not indicate tissue saturation. Tissue saturation causes diarrhea. The amount needed to get a urine reading is very much lower than the amount needed to cause diarrhea.
- The level of vitamin C in the urine is a good indication of the level in the tissues. If urinary levels are low, then so, too, will the tissue levels be low. High levels of excreted vitamin C are indications that the body's defenses are in good shape.
- Vitamin C is cheap.

Even a Little C Helps

According to new research, even if you drink only half a glass of orange juice or eat half a bowl of strawberries every day, you might not ever have a stroke. Reporting in the June 2002 issue of *Stroke: Journal of the American Heart Association*, Dr. Sudhir Kurl of the Research Institute of Public Health in Finland has concluded that not getting enough vitamin C in the foods you eat can increase your risk of stroke by more than twofold. And that risk is even higher for men who are overweight or have high blood pressure.

Kurl said his study is different from others conducted earlier that were inconclusive about the role of vitamin C in stroke prevention. This time, the Finnish researchers followed 2,419 men who were forty-two to sixty years old for about ten years, measuring the actual amount of vitamin C circulating in their blood—not just the amount of vitamin C they consumed from supplements and dietary sources as the previous studies did.

Vitamin C reduces the likelihood of a stroke in several ways. First, it reduces the effects of free radicals. Second, vitamin C helps protect the arteries against damage and lowers blood pressure and cholesterol levels.

Types of Vitamin C

It's important to point out there are a number of different forms of vitamin C. They are not all equal.

- As straight ascorbic acid, it is very acidic and may indeed lead to intense indigestion. In this form it is also difficult to dissolve in water; however, as a suspension it can be used as a mouthwash. Usually, vitamin C tablets are "buffered," which means they are in a non-acidic form.
- Most pro-vitamin C advocates warn that the calcium ascorbate form is not useful. Unfortunately, most on-the-shelf vitamin C pills are calcium ascorbate. A relatively new form of calcium ascorbate called Ester C is now on the market that claims to be four times more effective than normal vitamin C measured by its length of retention in the body and its bioavailabity. However, its effectiveness for cancer patients must remain in doubt.
- For cancer patients, sodium ascorbate is the preferred form. This can be prepared at home by mixing pure ascorbic acid and baking soda. The resulting powder can then be taken with any food; i.e., in cereal or on ice cream or as a suspension in a drink. It can also be bought in capsule or powder form. Others recommend a mixture of potassium and magnesium ascorbates. These, too, are available commercially.
- Only an ascorbate salt should be taken intravenously because ascorbic acid itself damages the veins and tissues into which it is injected. Linus Pauling, himself, and a number of other writers prefer to take L-ascorbic acid, fine crystals. This he took in orange juice or with a small amount of baking soda.
- In whatever form it is taken, it should, ideally, be divided into a number of equal doses and taken at regular intervals throughout the day. This is to maintain a high average daily level in the tissues.
- Vitamin C is best taken with an equal amount of bioflavonids, which are commonly found with vitamin C in nature. They are believed to protect vitamin C and to promote its absorption by the body of vitamin C. In combination they are also effective against oral herpes.

Food sources. Citrus juices and fruits, berries, tomatoes, potatoes, green and red peppers, broccoli and spinach. One cup (8 ounces) of reconstituted orange juice contains about 100 mg of vitamin C. *Side effects.* Taking excessive amounts of vitamin C (over 2,000 mg/day) might cause mild diarrhea. It may also interfere with stool tests for blood and other laboratory tests.

You should see your doctor before taking vitamin C if you have gout, kidney stones, sickle-cell anemia or iron storage disease. If you're pregnant or breast-feeding, don't take vitamin C in doses greater than the RDA for pregnant or breast-feeding women.

Vitamin E

Vitamin E is a fat-soluble vitamin, and a potent antioxidant that attaches directly to low-density lipoprotein (LDL) cholesterol (the "bad" cholesterol) in your blood and helps prevent damage from free radicals. Vitamin E is actually a general name for eight different compounds called "tocopherols" and "tocotrienols." There are four tocopherols called alpha, beta, gamma, and delta and there are four tocotrienols called alpha, beta, gamma, and delta.

Vitamin E comes in both a natural and synthetic form. Natural types of vitamin E are given the name d-alpha (or d-beta, etc.) or d-gamma, or d-delta) tocopherol. Synthetic vitamin E can be given the same name except there is a small "l" next to the little "d." So natural vitamin E would be "d-alpha tocopherol," and a synthetic type would be "dl-alpha tocopherol."

According to Mark A. Moyad, M.P.H. (Basic Science/Clinical Prostate Cancer Supplement Researcher & Lecturer, University of Michigan Medical-Urology/Oncology Dept.), recent studies, along with some past studies, have demonstrated that natural vitamin E is not only better absorbed by the human body than the synthetic type, but the liver does a better job of recognizing it and putting it into the blood.

Vitamin E and Our Hearts

Some studies show that it might prevent or slow progression of plaques forming within your artery walls (atherosclerosis) if you

Table 9.4 RDA and DRI for Vitamin E

Life Stage	Men and Women	Pregnant	Breastfeeding
Age 19+	22 IU* 33 IU†	–	–
Other	–	22 IU* 33 IU†	28 IU* 42 IU†

* Indicates vitamin E obtained from a natural source.
† Indicates vitamin E obtained from a synthetic source.

have heart disease or diabetes. However, other recent studies show no benefit from vitamin E supplements in high-risk heart patients.

Many Americans began taking vitamin E (now one of the top-selling supplements nationwide) a few years ago after studies suggested that it might protect against heart disease. In one study published in *Lancet* in 1996, men and women with cardiovascular disease who took the vitamin each day cut their risk of a second heart attack almost in half. In 1993, the *Journal of the National Cancer Institute* published findings from a five-year Chinese study that followed nearly thirty thousand adults. Those who took vitamin E supplements were 9 percent less likely to die during the study period.

The Cambridge Heart and Antioxidant study on two thousand people showed that 400–800 IU vitamin E per day is optimal for protection against cardiovascular disease, significantly reducing the risk of heart attack. The Harvard Nurses study, conducted on over eighty-seven thousand U.S. nurses showed that vitamin E can reduce the risk of coronary heart disease by 40 percent.

Many researchers have cautioned that more investigations were needed to confirm the power of vitamin E. But privately, some also admitted that they were taking a daily dose of the vitamin themselves, because the initial findings looked so good.

Then, in the January 20, 2000 issue of the *New England Journal of Medicine* reported the hype over vitamin E might be just that— hype. In a recent study, Canadian researchers tracked 2,545 women and 6,996 men aged fifty-five or older who took either vitamin E or a dummy pill. After five years, those taking the vitamin were no better off than those taking the dummy pill, suffering just as many heart attacks, strokes and deaths from cardiovascular disease. The findings, ironically, are part of a study called HOPE, or the Heart Outcomes Prevention Evaluation.

This wasn't the only study to cast a shadow over the vitamin's reputation. An Italian report published in *Lancet* in 2001, tested 300 IU of vitamin E against a placebo in a group of eleven thousand heart attack patients. Although the number of overall deaths related to cardiovascular disease for those taking the vitamin was lower, the number of second heart attacks in the same group was actually slightly higher. Neither of these numbers was, however, statistically significant, making it difficult to draw a firm conclusion.

New Starring Roles for Vitamin E

Despite the disappointing news, some heart specialists think it's still worth taking—especially by people who already have cardiovascular disease. Douglas Morris, M.D., Director of the Heart Center at Emory University in Atlanta, admits that he would still take vitamin E along with vitamin C, if he were diagnosed with heart disease. After all, vitamin E at doses of 800 IU or less a day has no known side effects. And some cardiologists are still recommending the vitamin to patients with heart disease. Moreover, other evidence suggests that vitamin E may provide additional important payoffs.

Research has found that vitamin E helps keep the immune system strong as we age. For instance, when researchers at Tufts University in Boston tested vitamin E capsules against placebos in healthy volunteers sixty-five or older, they found that those who took 200 IU per day showed a 65 percent increase in the activity of their immune cells in response to foreign substances. The vitamin E group also experienced a six-fold increase in antibodies to hepatitis-B vaccination—evidence that their immune systems were much stronger in creating defenses against the disease.

Higher doses of vitamin E may also delay or even prevent Alzheimer's disease. Patients with the illness who took the supplement were much less likely to be hospitalized than those who didn't, according to a 1997 study by physician Michael Grundman of the University of California at San Diego. "Vitamin E seemed to delay the onset of the worst symptoms of Alzheimer's," says Grundman, who is associate director of the Alzheimer's Disease Cooperative Study. "Because of its antioxidant property, it may work by blocking oxidative damage in the brain."

Some studies also suggested vitamin E may slow the progression of Parkinson's disease, enhance immunity in older adults, and help prevent prostate cancer, but more research is needed. A 2001 study indicates that supplementation with vitamin E, certain other antioxidants and zinc may slow the progression of age-related macular degeneration, but a doctor's supervision is important to determine proper doses to lower the risk of side effects.

Cure for Prostate Cancer?

A 1998 study published in the *Journal of the National Cancer Institute* suggests that alpha-tocopherol might reduce the risk of advanced prostate cancer. A placebo-controlled, double-blind trial carried out by Olli P. Heinonen and his colleagues at the University of Helsinki in Finland, studied 29,133 men ages fifty to sixty-nine. The subjects received alpha-tocopherol (50 IU daily), beta-carotene (20 mg daily), both supplements together, or a placebo. The treatments were continued for five to eight years.

Multivitamins generally contain about 30 IU of vitamin E, but single supplements most often have a minimum of 100 IU of vitamin E. The dose of 50 IU in the Finnish study is about five times the Recommended Dietary Allowance of vitamin E for men, and about three times what most people get from food.

Compared with the placebo group, the men taking only alpha-tocopherol developed 36 percent fewer prostate cancers. The men taking both supplements had a 16 percent lower incidence, while those taking only beta-carotene had a 20 percent higher incidence than the placebo group.

Combined, the two groups receiving alpha-tocopherol developed 32 percent fewer prostate cancers than the two groups that did not receive it. Their incidence of advanced cancer was 40 percent lower, and their mortality from prostate cancer was 41 percent lower. Researchers found these differences statistically significant.

However, they found alpha-tocopherol had no significant effect on the incidence of late-stage cancer. Nor did it affect survival time after diagnosis, indicating that once advanced cancer had developed, alpha-tocopherol did not influence its course.

These results suggest that vitamin E may help prevent prostate cancer from moving from the latent to the progressive stage. How it might do so is uncertain, but several mechanisms are possible. Its antioxidant properties may prevent free radical damage, or it may protect against cancer by increasing immunity. Vitamin E also has been reported to depress the activity of protein kinase-C, an enzyme that regulates cell proliferation.

Despite the striking results, this study has some potential sources of bias and must be interpreted cautiously. For one thing, the study was designed primarily to investigate alpha-tocopherol and beta-carotene in the prevention of lung cancer. Therefore, all the subjects were smokers.

Also—and I hope you can follow me here—since there is evidence that alpha-tocopherol may also reduce an enlarged prostate (known as BPH) men who take vitamin E would have fewer symptoms and would therefore be less likely to receive tests that might lead to cancer diagnosis. Also, it's suspected vitamin E supplements may also create other risks. Among those taking it in the study, there were sixty-six deaths from cerebral hemorrhage compared with forty-four such deaths among the men not taking vitamin E.

As you might suspect, further clinical trials are needed before vitamin E can be recommended for prostate cancer prevention.

Vitamin E should always be taken with a meal for better absorption and to prevent an upset stomach. Also, you should know that the following can decrease vitamin E blood levels:

- high level of vitamin A (from supplements)
- high intake of wheat bran
- high intake of pectin
- high intake of alcohol
- smoking

Also, you should be cautious about taking vitamin E if you have high blood pressure since it may cause an initial increase in your reading. You should also be careful if you're already taking anticoagulants or aspirin since vitamin E also can thin your blood.

John Hathcock, Ph.D., Director of Nutritional and Regulatory Science for the Council for Responsible Nutrition, says vitamin E, in all forms, is one of the safest of all vitamins. He has found no adverse effects have been demonstrated with alpha-tocopherol at intakes of 1,200 IU or more.

Although some studies on the benefits of vitamin E supplements appear promising, it's important to remember two things. First, when it comes to preventing heart disease, many of the benefits from vitamin E supplements can be achieved by exercising, eating a healthy diet and managing other risk factors, such as high blood pressure and high cholesterol. Second, there isn't enough evidence yet to recommend vitamin E pills for the general population.

Check with your doctor first before taking vitamin E if you're taking blood-thinning (anticoagulant) medications. Vitamin E can complicate the proper control of blood thinning. See your doctor before taking vitamin E if you have iron-deficiency anemia, bleeding or clotting problems, cystic fibrosis, intestinal problems or liver disease. If you're pregnant or breast-feeding, don't take vitamin E in doses greater than the RDA for pregnant or breast-feeding women.

Food sources. Foods rich in vitamin E include vegetable oils (particularly those from safflower, sunflower and cotton seeds), grains, and nuts. The leading sources of vitamin E in the U.S. diet include salad dressings and mayonnaise, margarine, cake, cookies, doughnuts, and eggs. To ingest 50 IU of vitamin E from such foods would mean also taking in a great deal of extra fat. And if you're shooting for 400 to 800 IU, you better like nuts a lot (and also own a wheelbarrow). Therefore, supplements are a good idea.

Side effects. In rare cases, people who take vitamin E may develop dizziness, fatigue, headache, weakness, abdominal pain, diarrhea, flu-like symptoms, nausea or blurred vision. At high doses (above 1,500 IU natural or 1,100 IU synthetic source/day), vitamin E can cause side effects that can include bleeding (especially for people on blood-thinning medications) and gastrointestinal complaints. However, in general, vitamin E is very well tolerated by most people.

Selenium

Selenium is an essential trace mineral and antioxidant. It helps keep the immune system and the thyroid gland working properly. Some studies indicate that cancer deaths, including lung, colorectal, and prostate cancers, are lower among people with higher selenium blood levels. Also, the incidence of non-melanoma skin cancer is significantly higher in areas of the United States with low soil selenium levels.

Selenium functions largely through an association with proteins, known as selenoproteins. Several of the selenoproteins are enzymes, which help prevent damage to cells in the body by oxidants, either from the environment or from those produced in normal metabolism.

Keshan disease is a disease of the heart muscle (cardiomyopathy) that occurs almost exclusively in children. It is the only human disease that is firmly linked to selenium deficiency. Although the disease does not occur in the selenium rich United States and Canada, it occurs with varying frequency in areas of China where the soil is severely selenium deficient and intakes are thus very low.

Since the importance of selenium in human nutrition was only demonstrated in 1979, not many studies have been conducted on the effect of selenium on chronic disease risk. However, results of two small studies indicate that selenium intakes above the RDA may have an anticancer effect in humans.

The effect of selenium supplementation on the recurrence of certain types of skin cancers was studied in seven dermatology clinics in the US from 1983 through the early 1990s.

Although selenium intakes of 200 mcg per day had no effect on the recurrence of non-melanoma skin cancer compared to the placebo, significantly lower rates of prostate, colon, and total cancer were found among those taking the selenium supplement. In another study, the risk of prostate cancer for men receiving 200 mcg per day of selenium was one-third that of men receiving a placebo.

Table 9.5 RDA and DRI for Selenium

Life Stage	Men and Women	Pregnant	Breastfeeding
Age 19+	55 mcg	–	–
Other	– –	60 mcg	70 mcg

In 2001, a large study was launched to determine if selenium and vitamin E could help protect against prostate cancer, but results will take several years. However, at this time, the National Academy of Sciences does not recommend taking selenium in doses greater than the Daily Value (DV) of 70 mcg a day.

Even newer research demonstrates a link between selenium and bladder cancer. A new study, published in the November 2002 issue of *Cancer Epidemiology, Biomarkers and Prevention*, found that ex-smokers with high levels of selenium had less risk of bladder cancer. However, this didn't hold true for current smokers or non-smokers. Why? The researchers believe this is because non-smokers have not exposed their bodies to the same oxidative stress that former smokers have, and current smokers are overwhelming any positive effects from selenium due to the toxic chemicals found in tobacco.

Chronic selenium toxicity is called selenosis. It has been reported in some population groups in China. The most frequently reported symptoms of selenosis are hair and nail brittleness. Other reported symptoms are gastrointestinal disturbances, skin rash, garlic breath odor (caused by the selenium compounds), fatigue, irritability, and nervous system abnormalities. Thus, adults consuming over the tolerable upper intake level (UL) of 400 mcg per day of selenium may be at risk of brittle hair and nails and other adverse effects.

See your doctor before taking selenium in doses above the DV of 70 mcg a day. The National Academy of Science recommends if you're pregnant or breast-feeding, avoid selenium intake greater than the RDA (60 mcg daily if pregnant and 70 mcg daily if breastfeeding).

Food sources. Milk, broccoli, cabbage, poultry, fish, seafood, organ meats and whole-grain products. One slice of whole-wheat bread contains 10 mcg of selenium.

Table 9.6 RDA and DRI for Zinc

Life Stage	Men	Women	Pregnant	Breastfeeding
Age 19+	11 mg	8 mg	–	–
Other	–	–	11 mg	12 mg

Side effects. Taking excessive amounts of selenium may cause hair and nail loss. Other symptoms include gastrointestinal disturbance, skin rash, fatigue, irritability, tooth decay and nervous system abnormalities.

Zinc

Zinc is an essential mineral that is found in almost every cell. It stimulates the activity of approximately one hundred enzymes, which are substances that promote biochemical reactions in your body. Zinc supports a healthy immune system and is needed for wound healing, helps maintain your sense of taste and smell, is needed for DNA synthesis, and sexual maturation. Zinc also supports normal growth and development during pregnancy, childhood, and adolescence.

Zinc has been recognized as an essential trace mineral for plants, animals and humans since the 1930s. The average adult body contains between 1.5 and 3 grams of zinc with approximately 60 percent of this in the muscles, 30 percent in the bones and 6 percent in the skin.

Zinc and Colds

The effect of zinc treatments on the severity or duration of cold symptoms is controversial. A 1996 study of over one hundred employees of the Cleveland Clinic indicated that zinc lozenges decreased the duration of colds by one-half, although no differences were seen in how long fevers lasted or the level of muscle aches. Other researchers examined the effect of zinc supplements on cold duration and severity in over four hundred randomized subjects.

In their first study, a virus was used to induce cold symptoms. The duration of illness was significantly lower in the group receiving zinc gluconate lozenges (providing 13.3 mg zinc) but not in the group receiving zinc acetate lozenges (providing 5 or 11.5 mg zinc). None of the zinc preparations affected the severity of cold symptoms in the first three days of treatment. In the second study, which examined the effects of zinc supplements on duration and severity of natural colds, no differences were seen between individuals receiving zinc and those receiving a placebo (sugar pill).

Some studies indicate that taking a daily multivitamin-mineral supplement containing zinc may increase immune response in older people. However, other studies have shown just the opposite—that zinc might weaken the immune status of older people. Until the effects of taking supplemental zinc are known, it's better not to exceed the Daily Value (DV) of 15 mg, although vegetarians may need more than the RDAs shown in the chart.

If you take zinc lozenges for a cold, stop taking them once your cold is gone. In addition, a 2001 study indicates that supplementation with zinc and certain antioxidants may slow the progression of age-related macular degeneration (AMD), but because a small percentage of participants had side effects, a doctor's supervision is important to determine proper doses.

Zinc and the Prostate

Many researchers believe zinc is critical for prostate health. Why? Zinc can reduce prostate problems such as swelling while boosting male virility. This is a highly controversial subject. Here's what proponents say.

The prostate needs ten times more zinc than any other organ in the body. In fact, this mineral is more concentrated in the prostate than in any other tissue. It makes sense that zinc is vital for preventing prostate problems, including BPH sufferers. In thwarting BPH, zinc, along with vitamin B6, not only inhibits the production of 5-alpha-reductase thus reducing the levels of DHT, which causes over production of prostate cells. It also helps the body dump excess DHT.

Zinc also acts to lower levels of another hormone, prolactin, which controls the development of testosterone in the prostate. When men reach their forties, prolactin levels tend to increase, which in turn causes production of more 5-alpha-reductase. Scientists believe that zinc controls secretion of prolactin by the pituitary gland. In fact, the combination of zinc and vitamin B6 is so effective in reducing prolactin levels that many researchers believe that a deficiency in either one might be a main cause of prostate enlargement. Increasing zinc levels therefore restricts the actions of the hormones and leads to a reduction in prostate size.

In several controlled studies, zinc has proven to actually reverse prostate enlargement. For instance, Irving Bush and Associates at Chicago's Cook County Hospital, tested the effect of zinc on patients with BPH symptoms. All patients reported symptomatic improvements, and 75 percent had noticeable shrinkage of the prostate.

In a 1996 study, researchers investigated the relationship between zinc and testosterone in forty normal men, aged from twenty to eighty. After twenty weeks of zinc restriction, they found lower testosterone in young men, while normal elderly men who took zinc supplements for six months had a marked increase in testosterone.

Zinc and Cancer

Zinc is also believed to reduce cancer risks. Zinc is required to utilize carotenes, and, therefore, may be cancer protective.

A good source for zinc is from animal and fishes as these high protein foods contain amino acids, which bind to zinc and make it more soluble. Specifically, good sources of zinc include liver, shellfish, oysters, meat, canned fish, hard cheese, whole grains, nuts, eggs and pulses. The zinc in grains is found mainly in the germ and bran coverings, so food refining and processing reduce the amount of zinc in food. For example, flour refining causes a 77 percent loss in zinc, rice refining causes a loss of 83 percent and processing cereals from whole grains causes an 80 percent loss.

Vegetables contain smaller amounts of zinc and also contain compounds such as phytates and oxalates, which bind zinc, leaving less available for absorption. Also, food additives and chemicals such as EDTA, which are used in food processing, reduce zinc absorption as do large amounts of textured vegetable protein.

Unfortunately, 90 percent of us consume diets deficient in zinc because most of the zinc in our food is lost in processing, or never exists in a substantial amount due to our nutrient-poor soils. Also, zinc does not store well in the body, and a reduction in dietary intake leads to deficiency fairly quickly. Excretion of zinc is mainly via the feces but some is lost in the urine. Excessive sweating can cause losses of up to 3 mg per day.

Thinking Zinc

Zinc is widely available as an over-the-counter dietary supplement. Specifically, zinc supplements, especially in the form of zinc picolinate or zinc citrate, might be beneficial in reducing the enlargement of the prostate and to reduce the symptoms.

If you supplement your diet with zinc, here are some important points to remember:

- Zinc supplements are available in various forms such as zinc gluconate, zinc sulfate, zinc picolinate or chelated zinc.
- Zinc supplements may be best taken first thing in the morning or two hours after meals. However, taking the supplements with meals helps to reduce nausea, which occurs in some people who take zinc on an empty stomach.
- Zinc and copper have related roles in many body functions and the balance between the two nutrients is important. If you regularly take zinc in doses of 25 mg or above it is wise to take 2 to 3 mg of copper to avoid imbalances in the copper-to-zinc ratio.
- Toxic effects of zinc are rare. High doses (around 200 mg) can cause abdominal pain, nausea and vomiting. Other symptoms include dehydration, lethargy, anemia and dizziness.

Don't take zinc if you have stomach or duodenal ulcers. See your doctor before taking zinc in doses above the Daily Value of 15 mg or if you're taking a calcium supplement or tetracycline drugs. Zinc may interfere with absorption of these medicines. If you're pregnant or breast-feeding, don't take zinc in doses greater than the RDA for pregnant or breast-feeding women.

On its own, the body has a hard time absorbing zinc. Deficiencies most often occurs when zinc intake is inadequate, when there are increased losses of zinc from the body, or when the body's requirement for zinc increases. Unless it is combined with vitamin B6, zinc cannot be converted into a form that is readily used by the prostate. Therefore, any therapy using zinc supplementation must also include adequate intake of vitamin B6.

Symptoms of zinc deficiency include the following:

- eczema on the face and hands
- hair loss

- diarrhea
- growth retardation
- delayed sexual maturation
- eye and skin lesions
- loss of the senses of taste and smell
- anemia
- poor appetite
- weight loss
- impaired conduction and nerve damage
- white spots on the nails
- apathy
- mental lethargy
- mental disorders
- susceptibility to infections
- delayed wound-healing
- impotence in men.

Since many of these symptoms are general and are associated with other medical conditions, do not assume they are due to a zinc deficiency.

You should know that zinc absorption decreases with age. People over sixty-five may absorb half as much zinc as those between twenty-five and thirty years old.

Food sources. Meat, fish, poultry, liver, eggs, milk, oysters, wheat germ and whole-grain products. A 3-ounce portion of lean sirloin contains 5 mg of zinc.

Side effects. Long-term, high doses of zinc (50 to 100 mg/day) lower high-density lipoprotein (HDL) cholesterol (the "good" cholesterol), suppress immune system function, and interfere with the absorption of copper, which may result in a condition known as microcytic anemia. Less severe side effects may include diarrhea, heartburn, nausea, vomiting and abdominal pain.

Try for Balance

Vitamins and minerals do not occur alone in nature. They always work together. This synergy and balance is vital in antioxidant activity. Vitamin E, for example, is regenerated by vitamin C and

supported by selenium. Also, vitamin E prevents lipid peroxida-
tion, but in the process becomes oxidized into a damaging toco-
pheroxyl radical. This process can be reversed by vitamin C.

On the other hand, while both vitamins C and E taken alone, can
prevent damaging oxidation of blood fats called lipids, which is
tied to cardiovascular disease, taking the two vitamins together
doesn't seem to give an added benefit. According to researchers at
Johns Hopkins University in Baltimore, a number of studies have
suggested that antioxidant vitamins like C and E may help ward off
oxidative damage and that these two vitamins may enhance each
others' protective powers. But much of this research has been in the
lab rather than in people, the authors of the study, published in the
September 2002 issue of the *American Journal of Clinical Nutrition*,
point out.

Although there is no solid evidence that high doses of single
antioxidant vitamins are really harmful, it is common sense not to
take too much of any one on their own. When we take vitamins and
minerals together in the proper balance, they will be more effective
at lower doses.

Also, when selecting a supplement for antioxidant protection,
look for optimum rather than RDA levels of essential nutrients.
Choose a combination of vitamin and plant antioxidants. When
selecting minerals, choose chelated minerals because these are
minerals combined with organic molecules that are absorbed via
active transport mechanisms in the small intestine. In other words,
they're easier for your body to absorb and use.

Why Aren't Carotenoids on the List?

You might be curious why there are no RDA/DRIs proposed for
the carotenoids, especially beta-carotene. According the National
Academy of Sciences, there's plenty of evidence showing higher
blood concentrations of beta-carotene and other carotenoids
obtained from foods lead to lower risks of several chronic diseases.
However, they say the evidence, although consistent, cannot be
used to establish a requirement for beta-carotene or total
carotenoid intake because the observed effects may be due to other
substances found in carotenoid-rich food, or to other factors related to increased fruit and vegetable consumption. "While there is

evidence that beta-carotene is an antioxidant in cell culture, its importance to health as an antioxidant is not yet adequately demonstrated," reports the NAS. "In the judgment of the experts who developed the report this data was not yet adequate on which to base a recommended intake."

Huh? To me, this is a cop-out. Couldn't the same argument be made about any beneficial nutrient? Can they be sure the benefits from vitamin A, or C, or selenium, for example, are not due to help from other nutrients, or simply by a person's choice to make sure they get the right nutrient through increased fruit and vegetable consumption?

Carotenoids consist of more than six hundred compounds that are found in some species of living organisms including animals, plants, and microorganisms. The most prevalent carotenoids in North American diets include the following: beta-carotene, alpha-carotene, lycopene, lutein, zeaxanthin and beta-cryptoxanthin.

In humans, the most important role of carotenoids is to act as a source of vitamin A in the diet. Carotenoids have been associated with various health effects such as decreased risk of macular degeneration of the eye and cataracts, decreased risk of some cancers, and decreased risk of some cardiovascular events.

By their own admission, the NAS recognizes higher consumption of carotenoid-containing fruits and vegetables and higher plasma concentrations of several carotenoids are associated with a lower risk of many different cancers, especially lung, oral cavity, pharyngeal, laryngeal, and cervical cancers.

There have never been any adverse effects other than carotenodermia reported from the consumption of beta-carotene or other carotenoids from food. Carotenodermia is characterized by a yellowish discoloration of the skin. It is considered harmless and is readily reversible when carotene ingestion is discontinued.

I don't think there's a sinister plot against carotenoids to keep them off the RDA/DRI list. I think it's simply because they, along with other important antioxidants (which I'll describe in the next chapter), don't fit in the government's neat little vitamin or mineral boxes. If that's the reason why—especially since these substances are so important—then I think the exclusion is a crying shame and a disservice to us all.

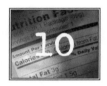

Antioxidants Not on the RDA/DRI List

If you've hunted for sound and complete nutritional information about antioxidants, you've probably discovered terms like "polyphenols," "caretonoids", "flavonoids," "isoflavones," "phytochemicals," and maybe even "nutraceuticals," "whole foods" or "functional foods." That is, if you read about nutrition in places other than the RDA/DRI reports.

Despite multiple volumes and thousands of pages, these terms are virtually absent from these tomes. Oh, I do think I saw mention of phytochemicals and the others in a few places in one or two volumes, but their significance, which should have been trumpeted on high, were mostly buried deep in nutritional techno-speak.

Despite a long standing belief and growing evidence that these and other substances can thwart diseases, they're not even listed on the RDA/DRI charts. Technically, they're not even considered nutrients. So, when the powers that be plot their antioxidant charts they include vitamins A, C, E, selenium and zinc, but leave out a whole slew of these other important compounds including beta-carotene. While these food components often accompany the better-known vitamins and minerals in foods, I firmly believe they deserve mention on their own. They're that important to our well-being.

Maybe you've heard claims these substances can ward off disease but you not really sure how or why. The terms do overlap and their distinctions can be cloudy. But, they're important enough—in fact they are so important in what they are and what they can do for us—their meaning and impact on our health should be clear to everyone. Alas, much too often they're not.

If I Were in Charge

If I were formulating the U.S. government's nutritional standards, beyond the scant few antioxidants on the RDA/DRIs list, I would feature phytochemicals front and center in terms of importance. And all of the polyphenols caretonoids, flavonoids, isoflavones, etc., etc., etc., would be listed on any chart I produced. They wouldn't be lost in thousands of pages, and I wouldn't allow or weight opinions from lobbyists and special interest groups. But they haven't asked me to participate. But by you picking up this book, I suspect you're looking for some guidance, at least indirectly. If that's the case, I'm happy to oblige.

I'm going to assume you haven't heard these terms and that you're curious what exactly they mean. Or maybe you have and aren't sure of their significance.

Here they are in a nutshell. Although this list isn't exhaustive by any means, at least you'll get a sense of the value of the most common antioxidants. Many of these terms overlap, and you'll find some of them in other lists of amino acids, enzymes and the like. It really doesn't matter where or how they're listed. What's important is their effect on our bodies. So here are, in my humble opinion, the most important:

Antioxidant. As a reminder, these help protect our bodies from the potentially harmful effects of free radicals, which can disrupt biological molecules and can damage tissue and cells in the body, and can contribute to the development of diseases including cancer and heart disease.

Phytochemicals/phytonutrients. These are plant chemicals that contain protective, disease-preventing compounds. Phytochemicals are non-nutritive, which doesn't mean much in the grand scheme of things, except they can't be classified as either vitamins or minerals.

Carotenoids (or carotenes). These compounds are the natural colorings in fruits and vegetables that can boost our immune systems and can help protect our bodies from cancer. (Carotenoids are oil soluble.)

Polyphenols. These natural phytochemicals are found in tea leaves, most fruits and vegetables and in vitamins and minerals. Often this term is used interchangeably with flavonoids.

Flavonoids (also known as bioflavonoids). Flavonoids are natural chemicals found abundantly in fruit and vegetables. Chemically they are known as polyphenols and are water soluble.

Isoflavones. These phytonutrients are related to flavonoids and are found in soy, chick peas and other legumes. Isoflavones work as enzyme inhibitors, thereby decreasing cancer cell growth.

Here are some other terms you may have heard:

Whole foods. Whole foods are natural, unprocessed foods like fresh fruits, vegetables, and grains (still in their original state with all their vital nutrients intact).

Nutraceutical. Nutraceuticals are specific chemical compounds in food that might aid in preventing disease promote health. They are naturally occurring dietary substances that can be sold as "dietary supplements."

Functional foods. Any food or food ingredient that may provide a health benefit beyond the traditional nutrients it contains can be called a functional food.

Whole foods are the natural carriers for the nutrients your body needs—complete with the enzymes needed to break them down. Your body recognizes these foods and knows how to digest and distribute the nutrients within them.

Food products that have been heat processed, stripped, separated, or preserved with chemicals are not whole foods. Most of the nutrients originally found in these foods have been lost due to over processing—fiber is stripped out, vitamins and minerals have been dissipated through heat or chemical processing, and living enzymes and amino acids have been destroyed. The few nutrients left in foods after processing are stripped of their original enzymes, identity, and also lose most of their effectiveness.

Many recent, well-documented studies show diets rich in whole foods increase your body's resistance to disease and increase your longevity. In 1999, the American Institute for Cancer Research found that more than one-third of Americans were lacking in necessary nutrients due to lack of whole foods. People who consistently eat suggested levels of these foods are at lower risk of high blood pressure, cancer, diabetes, heart disease and stroke.

It's believed the first person to use the term *nutraceutical* was Stephen de Felice, M.D., director of New York's Foundation for Innovation in Medicine. According to Paul Lachance, Ph.D., Nutrition and Food Science Professor and Director of the Nutraceuticals Institute at Rutgers University, nutraceutical refers to the naturally derived, bioactive compounds in foods that have health benefits. An example of a nutraceutical would be lycopene, the naturally occurring compound in tomatoes that help fight against certain cancers.

Functional foods are foods that contain nutraceuticals and provide this extra health benefit in addition to the nutrients normally found in the item. For example, both tomatoes (also considered a whole food), and tomato products with lycopene, are considered functional foods. Another example of a functional food would be orange or grapefruit juice fortified with calcium for bone-strength.

Phytochemicals

Phytochemical is a more recent evolution of the term *nutraceutical* emphasizing the plant source of most of these protective, disease-preventing compounds. Research in this area is expanding rapidly because it appears that phytonutrients offer the best protection we know of against the diseases that plague us today. More than four thousand phytochemicals have been identified so far, but only about 150 have been intensively studied, according to the University of California Berkeley's *Wellness Letter*.

A true nutritional role for phytochemicals is becoming more probable every day as research uncovers more of their remarkable benefits. In fact, the term phytonutrient better describes the compounds' "quasi-nutrient" status. Someday, phytochemicals may indeed be classified as essential nutrients. We might even call them "vitamins." Who knows?

Studies show as we move away from the diet of our ancestors we are more susceptible to "modern" diseases. Scientists have studied long-existing societies such as the centenarian tribes that live in remote villages in the Andes Mountains and who never wavered from their traditional dietary practices. These people have been reported to live extraordinarily long lives that are free of such illnesses as cancer, heart disease and arthritis.

By contrast, researchers have examined epidemiological evidence from modern societies for clues to the diet-disease connection. On the basis of such studies, biochemical researchers have pinpointed certain phytochemicals—found only in whole grains and fresh fruits and vegetables that aid the body in maintaining health and combating disease.

Phytochemicals and Cancer

Research continues to discover and confirm that cancer is a largely avoidable disease. It is estimated that more than two-thirds of cancer might be prevented through lifestyle modification, with nearly one-third of these cancers eliminated by improvements in diet. While the U.S. Dietary Guidelines do discuss the need for changes of the American diet of high-fat, low-fiber foods to low-fat, high-fiber foods and more fruits and vegetables, personally I don't think they emphasize this link enough.

By now we should all know eating fruits and vegetables reduces the risk of many cancers. One major prevention strategy has been the "5 A Day for Better Health" program sponsored by the National Cancer Institute (NCI), encouraging the public to include more fruits and vegetables in its diet. But do we?

How many of us follow the American Cancer Society's guidelines for nutrition and cancer prevention. These guidelines, which are similar to the Dietary Guidelines for Americans, include the following:

- Choose most of the foods you eat from plant sources.
- Limit your intake of high-fat foods, particularly from animal sources.
- Be physically active. Achieve and maintain a healthy weight.
- Limit consumption of alcoholic beverages if you drink at all.

The guideline stating to "choose most of the foods you eat from plant sources" has been recognized for years as important for good health. But do you see it publicized on television between ads for fast food or heartburn remedies? Neither have I, but they should be.

More and more top-flight research is describing properties, specifically naturally occurring compounds contained in fruits, vegetables, grains, legumes, seeds, licorice root, soy, green tea and other foods. Chemical compounds found in these foods are being recognized for their potential for protection against not just cancer but cardiovascular problems and other diseases.

To date, more than nine hundred different phytochemicals have been identified as components of food, and many more continue to be discovered all the time. It is estimated that there may be more than one hundred different phytochemicals in just one serving of vegetables. It's believed there are hundreds of other phytochemicals existing in foods haven't been discovered yet.

As early as 1980, the National Cancer Institute Chemoprevention Program of the Division of Cancer Prevention and Control began evaluating phytochemicals for safety, efficacy, and applicability for preventing and treating diseases. Researchers have long known that there are phytochemicals present for protection in plants. But it was only recently that health professionals and scientists started recommending them for protection against human disease.

Why Phytochemicals Are Valuable

At one time, some of these compounds found in fruits and vegetables were classified as vitamins:

- Flavonoids were known as vitamin P.
- Cabbage factors (glucosinolates and indoles) were for some time called vitamin U.
- Ubiquinone was vitamin Q.

Tocopherol somehow stayed on the list as vitamin E. Vitamin designation was dropped for the other nutrients because specific deficiency symptoms could not be established.

Recent research, however, has enabled scientists to group phytonutrients into classes on the basis of similar protective functions as well as individual physical and chemical characteristics of the molecules.

Table 10.1 The Most Commonly Studied Phytochemicals

Food	Phytochemicals
Allium vegetables (garlic, onions, chives, leeks)	Allyl sulfides
Cruciferous vegetables (broccoli, cauliflower, cabbage, Brussels sprouts, kale, turnips, bok choy, kohlrabi)	Indoles/glucosinolates Sulfaforaphane Isothiocyanates/thiocyanates Thiols
Solanaceous vegetables (tomatoes, peppers)	Lycopene
Umbelliferous vegetables (carrots, celery, cilantro, parsley, parsnips)	Carotenoids Phthalides Polyacetylenes
Compositae plants (artichoke)	Silymarin
Citrus fruits (oranges, lemons, grapefruit)	Monoterpenes (limonene) Carotenoids
Glucarates Other fruits (grapes, berries, cherries, apples, cantaloupe, watermelon, pomegranate)	Ellagic acid Phenols Flavonoids (quercetin)
Beans, grains, seeds (soybeans, oats, barley, brown rice, whole wheat, flax seed) Protease inhibitors	Flavonoids (isoflavones) Phytic acid Saponins

Table 10.1 continued

Food	Phytochemicals
Herbs, spices (ginger, mint, rosemary, thyme, oregano, sage, basil, tumeric, caraway, fennel)	Gingerols Flavonoids Monoterpenes (limonene)
Licorice root Green tea Polyphenols	Glycyrrhizin Catechins

Although phytochemicals are not presently classified as nutri-ents—compounds necessary for sustaining life—they have been identified as containing properties for aiding in disease preven-tion. Phytochemicals are associated with the prevention and/or treatment of at least four of the leading causes of death in the United States—cancer, diabetes, cardiovascular disease, and hyper-tension. They are involved in many processes including ones that help prevent cell damage, prevent cancer cell replication, and decrease cholesterol levels.

According to the American Cancer Society's *Cancer Facts & Figures 1997,* the cost of cancer to society was estimated to be about $104 billion in that year, and it certainly isn't getting any cheaper. With health care costs being a major issue today, it would be cost effective to continue the research needed to help promote the awareness and consumption of phytochemicals as a prevention strategy for the public—at least to my way of thinking.

Following is a look at each of the phytonutrient classes (or phy-tochemicals if you're a stickler for details). It is fairly confusing to identify in which class a phytonutrient belongs, but this informa-tion is important to know because each class offers a unique kind of protection for the body. Suffice it to say, all of them are impor-tant. (Don't fret. I'm not going to cover all four thousand phto-chemicals; I don't want to bury what's important.)

Terpenes

Terpenes such as those found in green foods, soy products and grains comprise one of the largest classes of phytonutrients. The most intensely studied terpenes are carotenoids—as evidenced by the many recent studies on beta-carotene. The terpenes function as antioxidants, protecting lipids, blood and other body fluids from assault by free radical oxygen species including singlet oxygen, hydroxyl, peroxide and superoxide radicals. Terpenoids are dispersed widely throughout the plant kingdom, protecting plants from the same reactive oxygen species that attack human cells.

Carotenoids

This terpene subclass consists of bright yellow, orange and red plant pigments found in vegetables such as tomatoes, parsley, oranges, pink grapefruit, spinach and red palm oil that work together to help knock out free radicals. We even find carotenoids lending bright colors to animals; flamingos owe their color to carotenoids, as do shellfish. Egg yolks are yellow because of carotenoids that protect the unsaturated fats in the yolk. There are more than six hundred carotenoid compounds found in animals, plants and microorganisms.

The most prevalent carotenoids in North American diets include the following: beta-carotene, alpha-carotene, lycopene, lutein, zeaxanthin and beta-cryptoxanthin.

Most people think of this family of phytonutrients as being precursors to vitamin A, but fewer than 10 percent are. Only three of the above most prevalent carotenoids—beta-carotene, alpha-carotene and beta-cryptoxanthin—are converted to vitamin A. They are referred to as provitamin A carotenoids. Of these, beta-carotene is the most active.

Beta-carotene

Probably the best known carotenoid is beta-carotene. A good source of Vitamin A, it is found in carrots, cantaloupe, pumpkin, sweet potatoes and tomatoes.

Some studies indicate that diets high in beta-carotene and other carotenoids obtained from food are associated with a lower risk of several chronic diseases such as heart disease and some cancers. It's believed beta-carotene acts as a cancer preventive, by inhibiting the formation of free radicals. However, this effect may be due to other substances found in carotenoid-rich foods, not only beta-carotene.

Several well-designed studies have found that supplements of beta-carotene offer no protection against heart disease. Three large clinical trials found that beta-carotene supplements did not protect against cancer. Two studies found an increased risk of lung cancer among smokers who took beta-carotene supplements, and one found an increased risk of prostate cancer among men who took beta-carotene supplements and also drank alcohol. A large Finnish study found that daily supplements of beta-carotene had no effect on the prevalence of cataracts.

A recent study indicates that a small amount of beta-carotene taken with certain other antioxidants and zinc may slow the progression of age-related macular degeneration (AMD) the most common cause of sight loss in people over sixty-five.

Other members of the carotenoid family include the following:

Alpha-carotene. (From carrots and pumpkins)
Lutein. (In dark-green, leafy vegetables like spinach and collard greens.) Helps clear away free radicals caused by harmful ultraviolet rays. It also slows macular degeneration.
Lycopene. (In tomatoes) Lutein can help keep eyes healthy. Lycopene may prevent cancer, stroke and sun damage to the body.
Xanthophyll. (Yellow pigment in plants and egg yolks.)
Zeaxanthin. (Watercress, Swiss chard, spinach, okra, chicory, and the yellow pigment in corn. Protects the eye from macular degeneration due to free radical damage.

Alpha-carotene provides 50 percent to 54 percent of the antioxidant activity of beta-carotene. (Another carotene, epsilon-carotene, has 42 percent to 50 percent as much.) These carotenes, along with lycopene and lutein, which do not convert to vitamin A, seem to offer protection against lung, colorectal, breast, uterine and prostate cancers. Carotenes are "tissue-specific" in their protection, meaning for maximum overall protection, you should try to take them all together.

Carotenes also enhance immune response and protect skin cells against UV radiation. Additionally, they "spare" the detoxification enzymes in the liver that we rely on to safely eliminate pollutants and toxins from the body.

The xanthophyll type of carotenoids also include many interesting molecules. One xanthophyll, canthaxantin, was popular as a tanning pill a few years ago. It migrates to the skin and protects it from sunlight. Other important xanthophylls are cryptoxanthin, zeaxanthin and astaxanthin.

Xanthophylls are important because they appear to protect vitamin A, vitamin E and other carotenoids from oxidation. Evidence is emerging that xanthophylls are protective of specific body tissues. Cryptoxanthin, for example, may be highly protective of vaginal, uterine and cervical tissues.

Lutein Also Aids the Arteries

Besides aid for aging eyes, a University of Southern California (USC) study shows lutein can help prevent the hardening and narrowing of arteries that can lead to a heart attack or stroke. In the study, the researchers looked at the impact of lutein on atherosclerosis in carotid (neck) arteries. Carotid artery thickness is an indication of atherosclerosis throughout the body. It can lead to a heart attack or stroke.

The results of the eighteen-month study of nearly five hundred middle-aged men and women showed those who had the highest levels of lutein in their blood also showed the least thickening in their artery walls. "The most important information for consumers is that a diet rich in vegetables may be protective against the disease that leads to most heart attacks and strokes," said researcher James H. Dwyer, Ph.D., professor of preventive medicine, Keck School of Medicine, at USC. The study appears in the June 19, 2001 issue of *Circulation: Journal of American Heart Association*.

Learn to Like Lycopene

Besides tomatoes, lycopene is found in carrots, spinach, papaya, guava, rosehip, watermelon and pink grapefruit. Lycopene is deposited in the liver, lungs, prostate gland, colon and skin. Its concentration in tissues tends to be higher than all other carotenoids.

Research shows lycopene can be absorbed more efficiently by the body after it's processed into ketchup, juice, sauce and paste since the cooking temperature used in processing converts it to a more absorbable form. Remember, though, many of these processed foods have additives, including sugar. Recently, Heinz came out with an organic ketchup, which tastes different than typical ketchup. In my opinion, it tasted more like tomatoes than other ketchups.

In a six-year Harvard study, the diets of more than forty-seven thousand men were studied. Of forty-six fruits and vegetables evaluated, only the tomato products (which contain large quantities of lycopene) showed a measurable relationship to reduced prostate cancer risk. As consumption of tomato products increased, levels of lycopene in the blood increased, and the risk for prostate cancer decreased. The study also showed that the heat processing of tomatoes and tomato products increases lycopene's bioavailability.

In another Harvard study, of nearly one thousand postmenopausal women researchers found those with the highest blood levels of lycopene were about one-third less likely to develop heart disease when compared with those who had the lowest levels. Half the women in the Harvard study had suffered a heart attack or developed serious heart complications; half had no heart problems. All had their blood lycopene level measured when the study began in 1992. Lead author Howard Sesso said the statistical analysis showed that when other risk factors for heart disease were taken into account, women whose lycopene levels were highest had a 34 percent reduction in heart disease risk, compared with those whose levels were lowest.

Limonoids

This terpene subclass, found in citrus fruit peels, appears to be specifically directed to protection of lung tissue. In one study, a standardized extract of d-limonene, pinene, and eucalyptol were effective in clearing congestive mucus from the lungs of patients with chronic obstructive pulmonary disease.

Limonoids might also act as specific chemopreventive agents. In animal studies, results suggest that the chemotherapeutic activity of limonoids helps activate detoxification enzymes in the liver.

Phytosterols

Phytosterols (often abbreviated to just sterols), occur in most plant species. They are plant compounds with chemical structures similar to that of cholesterol—the main animal sterol.

Although green and yellow vegetables contain significant amounts, their seeds concentrate the sterols. Most of the research on these valuable phytonutrients has been done on the seeds of pumpkins, yams, soy, rice and herbs. Phytosterols compete with dietary cholesterol for uptake in the intestines. They have demonstrated the ability to block the uptake of cholesterol (to which they are structurally related) and to facilitate its excretion from the body. Cholesterol has long been implicated as a significant risk factor in cardiovascular disease. Are other dietary factors important as well?

To answer this question, a research team in Los Angeles conducted a study to test the importance of other dietary factors in modifying the risk of cholesterol levels. They compared the diets of 169 Seventh Day Adventists (vegans, lacto-ovo and non-vegetarians) with general population non-vegetarians all living in Los Angeles in the mid 1980s. They found the ratio between dietary plant phytosterols and cholesterol was significantly lower in SDA vegetarians as compared to non-vegetarians. The importance of this study underlies the fact that cholesterol, per se, is not the only marker of risk for cardiovascular disease and that its ratio with other modifying dietary components may be a better measure of risk.

Other investigations have revealed that phytosterols block the development of tumors in colon, breast and prostate glands. What mechanisms cause this to occur are not well understood, but we do know that phytosterols appear to alter cell membrane transfer in tumor growth and reduce inflammation.

Beta-sitosterol is one of several plant sterols found in almost all plants. High levels are found in rice bran, wheat germ, corn oils, and soybeans. As one of several phytosterols, beta-sitosterol, alone as well as in combination with similar plant sterols, is known to lessen inflammation and block the accumulation of cholesterol in the prostate gland. The compound, however, does not appear to alter the size of the prostate. It has also been tested to block absorption of cholesterol in the whole body.

As with any substance taken to treat a disease, consult your doctor for guidance about taking beta-sitosterol for high cholesterol or prostate as a fairly high dose of the substance is needed to control the ailments. A doctor should always examine prostate problems, before you start taking beta-sitosterol so as to rule out other, more serious conditions, including prostate cancer.

Flavonoids

Flavonoids (also known as bioflavonoids) have potent antioxidant properties and can reduce oxidation of low-density lipoproteins, the harmful type of cholesterol. Like their better-known chemical cousins, the carotenes, flavonoids are plant pigments, creating a rainbow of colors. In addition, many flavonoids and carotenes function as antioxidants and protect plants from damaging free radicals. Flavonoids enhance the effects of vitamin C. As I mentioned earlier, they were once lumped together as vitamin P.

Besides apples and onions, flavonoids are also present in red wine, beer, ale, stout and tea. Researchers have identified more than four thousand of them in plants and believe there might be as many as twenty thousand found in nature.

Flavonoids act against allergies, inflammation, free radicals, toxins, microbes, ulcers, viruses and tumors. Flavonoids also inhibit specific enzymes. For example, flavonoids block the angiotensin-converting enzyme (ACE) that raises blood pressure. By blocking the "suicide" enzyme cyclooxygenase that breaks down prostaglandins, they stop blood platelets from sticking together and reduce the risk of a clot. Flavonoids also protect the vascular system and strengthen the capillaries that carry oxygen and essential nutrients to all cells.

Additionally, flavonoids block the enzymes that produce estrogen, thus reducing the risk of estrogen-induced cancers. One way they do this is by blocking estrogen synthsase, an enzyme that works overtime in binding estrogen to receptors in several organs.

They might also stabilize nucleic acid, thus reducing the potential risk of cancer. Flavonoids help the immune system to function better, and they might also help prevent the development of Alzheimer's disease.

Flavonoids also appear to retard development of cataracts in individuals with diabetes. Cataracts can be a complication of diabetes because diabetics, unable to metabolize sugar normally, build up damaging levels of "alcohol sugars." These in turn cause clouding of the lens of the eye (cataract). It is suspected flavonoids prevent cataracts by blocking aldose-reductase, a digestive enzyme, which can convert the sugar galactose into the potentially harmful form of galacticol. Here is a partial listing of the better known flavonoids:

Catechins, gallic acids. Catechins differ slightly in chemical structure from other flavonoids, but share their chemoprotective properties. The most common catechins are gallic esters, named epicatechin (EC), epicatechin gallate (ECG), and epigallocatechin gallate (EGCG). All are found in green tea, *Camellia sinensis*, and are thought to be responsible for the protective benefits of this beverage.

Smaller amounts of catechins are also in black tea, grapes, wine and chocolate. Due to their potent antioxidant capabilities, catechins, often referred to as "tea flavonoids," are being investigated for their ability to prevent cancer and heart disease. In experimental models, catechins show a wide range of protective effects, including cardioprotective, chemoprotective, and anitmicrobial properties.

Although black tea also has flavonoids, it seems to be green tea (unfermented) that has the higher amount of catechins. Green tea has about 27 percent catechins, with oolong tea (partially fermented) having about 23 percent, and black tea (fermented) at approximately 4 percent catechins. Researchers speculate that green tea's higher concentration of catechins is due to the way it is processed. Green tea harbors important compounds that may be reduced in black tea during the drying and fermentation process that produces black tea.

Resveratrol. Table grapes, like red wine and red grape juice, contain the phytochemical resveratrol. Found primarily in the skin of grapes, resveratrol has been found in preliminary studies to fight breast, liver and colon cancers. Resveratrol is also believed to play a role in the reduction of heart disease and has been shown to exhibit anti-inflammatory properties, according to the California Table Grape Commission. Table grapes also contain the phytochemicals quercetin, anthocyanin and catechin.

Proanthocyanidins or anthocyanidins. These highly specialized bioflavonoids have been extensively studied since the late 1960s for their powerful vascular wall strengthening properties and free radical scavenging activity.

Proanthocyanidins are also known under several other names, others among the most common are OPC, pycnogenols, and leukocyanidins. Proanthocyanidins are found in high concentrations from such sources as bilberry, cranberries, grape skins, grape seeds, pine bark, lemon tree bark, and hazel nut tree leaves. The two most common and richest known sources are grape seed extract and pine bark extract.

Carotenoids and Flavonoids?

It's very easy to get these two confused. The biggest difference between the two is that flavonoids are water soluble, whereas carotenes are oil soluble.

Phenols

These phytonutrients comprise a large class that has been the subject of extensive research as a disease preventive. Phenols protect plants from oxidative damage and perform the same function for humans. Blue, blue-red and violet colorations seen in berries, grapes and purple eggplant are due to their phenolic content. Bilberries, for example, are high in phenolic anthocyanidins and are red in color. The outstanding phytonutrient feature of phenols is their ability to block specific enzymes that cause inflammation. They also modify the prostaglandin pathways and thereby protect blood platelets from clumping.

Polyphenols

Polyphenols are the antioxidant flavonoid compounds found in green tea, fruits, fruit juices and alcoholic beverages such as beer and wine. Close to 40 percent of a green tea leaf is made of polyphenols. In tea, the chemicals are often referred to as tannins, which give tea the slightly bitter taste—especially when left to brew for a long time. Again, they are often described as flavonoids, although technically polyphenols present in plant materials are divided into two groups: either phenolic acids or flavonoids. Polyphenols occur naturally in many fruits as a natural color pigment and give characteristic colors of most fruits. They are natural substrates of enzymes called polypheoloxidases, which catalyze enzymatic browning. Polyphenols also are responsible for the haze formation and loss of clarity during the storage of clear juices and concentrates. In citrus juices, polyphenols cause bitterness, which is considered as one of the important problem of citrus juice processing.

Anthocyanidins

This group of flavonoids deserves special attention. Technically known as "flavonals," anthocyanidins provide crosslinks or "bridges" that connect and strengthen the intertwined strands of collagen protein. Collagen is the most abundant protein in the body, making up soft tissues, tendons, ligaments and bone matrix. Its great tensile strength depends on preservation of its crosslinks.

Anthocyanidins, being water soluble, also scavenge free radicals they encounter in tissue fluids. This is a powerful ability especially beneficial for athletes and others who exercise, because heavy exercise generates large amounts of free radicals.

Thiols

Phytonutrients of this sulfur-containing class are present in garlic and cruciferous vegetables (i.e., cabbage, turnips and members of the mustard family). Thiols have numerous functions, including a central role in coordinating the antioxidant defense network and overcoming oxidative stress during exercise.

Glucosinolates

Found in cruciferous vegetables, glucosinolates are powerful activators of liver detoxification enzymes. They also regulate white blood cells and cytokines. White blood cells are the scavengers of the immune system and cytokines act as "messengers," coordinating the activities of all immune cells.

Dithiolthiones and sulforaphane are protective of specific tissues. Their actions involve blocking enzymes that promote tumor growth, particularly in the breast, liver, colon, lung, stomach and esophagus.

Researchers have also found that sulforaphane, found in broccoli and broccoli sprouts, also kills *H. pylori*, the bacteria believed to be responsible for most ulcers and stomach cancers. It also appears to overcome antibiotic-resistant strains of bacteria.

Allylic Sulfides

Garlic and onions are the most potent members of this thiol subclass, which also includes leeks, shallots and chives. The allylic sulfides in these plants are released when the plants are cut or smashed. Once oxygen reaches plant cells, various bio-transformation products are formed. Each of these appears to have tissue specificity. As a group, allylic sulfides appear to possess antimutagenic and anticarcinogenic properties as well as immune and cardiovascular protection. They also appear to offer anti-growth activity for tumors, fungi, parasites, cholesterol and platelet/leukocyte adhesion factors.

Garlic and onions, like their cruciferous relatives, can also activate liver detoxification enzyme systems. Specific allylic sulfides block the activity of toxins produced by bacteria and viruses.

Indoles

This subclass includes phytonutrients that interact with vitamin C, which is not surprising since the vegetables that contain indoles also contain significant amounts of vitamin C. Indole complexes bind chemical carcinogens and activate detoxification enzymes, mostly in the gastrointestinal tract. The bio-transformation products of indoles are formed when they are acted on by stomach acid. The most active product is "ascorbigen," considered to be an active vitamin C "metabolite."

Isoprenoids

Isoprenoids neutralize free radicals in a unique way. They have a long carbon side-chain, which they use to anchor themselves into fatty membranes. Any free radicals that are attached to lipid (fat) membranes are quickly grabbed and passed off to other antioxidants.

Tocotrienols and Tocopherols

Tocotrienols naturally occur in grains and palm oil along with their cousins, tocopherols. Tocotrienols appear to inhibit breast cancer cell growth, whereas tocopherols do not exhibit this effect. Researchers have observed that the biologic functions of tocopherols and tocotrienols appear unrelated. Tocotrienols have been most studied, however, for their cholesterol lowering effects.

Lipoic Acid and Coenzyme Q10

Lipoic acid and coenzyme Q10 (often called co Q10) are important antioxidants that work to extend the effects of other antioxidants. In terms of research, lipoic acid is relatively new. Of course, no phytonutrient is actually new; it's only our understanding of them that's new.

Both lipoic acid and co Q10 have important roles in energy production. It is an efficient "hydroxyl radical quencher," and scavenges peroxyl, ascorbyl and chromanoxyl radicals. It also enhances both vitamin E and vitamin C. Lipoic acid also plays an important role in liver detoxification.

By thirty-five years of age and beyond, there are decreasing amounts of co Q10 available to the cellular systems that need it. And herein lies its value as a key to retarding the aging process. To the extent that any cell suffers from too little co Q10, the work of that cell is hindered.

Coenzyme Q10 is not widely known in the U.S. In Japan, as many as ten million people—nearly 10 percent of the entire country's population—take co Q10 on a daily basis. (In the U.S., so far, it has mostly extended the lifespans of some very fortunate laboratory animals.)

Hundreds of university studies, both here and abroad, have shown it can boost the immune system, relieve angina, protect against heart attacks, normalize heart rhythm, lower blood pressure, increase the strength of the heart, and assist in weight reduction. In a study reported in the October 2002 edition of the *Archives of Internal Medicine*, it was discovered co Q10 can slow the progression of the neurological illness Parkinson's disease.

In the study, Dr. Clifford W. Shults of the University of California-San Diego and colleagues found that Parkinson's patients have reduced levels of coenzyme Q10 in their mitochondria. This led the researchers to investigate whether the antioxidant would be useful in treating the disease. They found the progression of Parkinson's disease was significantly slower in people taking the highest dose of coenzyme Q10.

During the first twenty years of life co Q10 is manufactured at optimal levels but the ability to synthesize it declines with age, so that as we grow older we gradually develop a deficiency of it. If the cell in question happens to be an immune system cell, for example, the immune system will not function optimally, and infections and allergies will be more likely. If the cell is a neuron (nerve cell) the energy necessary for nerve impulse conduction will not be available. If it is a cell of the liver, kidney, lung, adrenal, pancreas, etc., those glands, organs and tissues will function less effectively. Daily co Q10 supplementation will prevent this erosion of optimal functioning and the premature aging that always accompanies it.

Isoflavones

Packed in every soybean are estrogen-like molecules, called isoflavones, which are believed to fight heart disease, osteoporosis, cancer and other diseases. Isoflavones, which are part of the phytoestrogen (or plant estrogen) family, function much like flavonoids in that they effectively block enzymes that promote tumor growth.

Based on just some of the latest findings in 2000, the Food and Drug Administration gave food makers permission to extol soy's cholesterol-lowering prowess on package labels.

Soy's three best-known compounds are the following:

Genistein. Genistein is a chemical compound found only in soybeans. Dr. Lothar Schweigerer at Heidelberg University discovered genistein blocks an event called angiogenesis, the growth of new blood vessels that nourish malignant tumors. Once a tumor grows beyond a millimeter, it must foster the growth of new blood vessels into it in order to become malignant and life threatening. By inhibiting blood vessel growth, genistein may keep new tumors from growing beyond harmless dimensions and eventually lead to the shrinking of the tumor. Genistein has also been shown to prevent bone loss in animals.

Pueraria. Pueraria has gained popularity as an aid for alcohol drinkers because it appears to alter the activity of alcohol detoxification enzymes, namely the speed at which alcohol dehydrogenase converts alcohol into aldehydes. The result is a lowered tolerance for alcohol and reduction of the pleasure response to drinking it.

Daidzein. Also found in soy, daidzein enhances bone formation leading scientists to believe it might prevent and treat osteoporosis.

Numerous studies show that eating soy may help prevent heart disease, endometriosis and even osteoporosis in women, said Larrian Gillespie, M.D., author of *The Menopause Diet* and *The Goddess Diet*. (*Note:* If you think you may have any of these conditions, see your doctor before making any substantive changes to your diet.)

Isoflavones and Cholesterol

Soy's biggest impact could be on cholesterol levels, according to a large number of studies. One study published in the December 1998 issue of the *American Journal of Clinical Nutrition* found that men who ate a low-fat diet and relied on soy as their main protein source for five weeks saw their "bad" (LDL) cholesterol levels decrease by as much as 14 percent and their "good" (HDL) levels increase by as much as 8 percent. Men who ate a low-fat diet but instead relied on meat as protein also saw their cholesterol levels significantly improve, though not as much as the soy-eaters. And eating soy helps replace animal products, which are loaded with saturated fats and cholesterol, says nutritionist Mark Messina, Ph.D., author of *The Simple Soybean and Your Health*.

When you switch from eating a cheeseburger to a soy burger, for example, you get a double benefit: you're not eating the large amounts of saturated fat and cholesterol found in the greasy cheeseburger and you're getting additional benefits from the soy protein itself.

Evidence that soy can lower cholesterol is so strong the Food and Drug Administration now allows the claim on food labels. (The FDA says: "25 grams of soy protein a day, as part of a diet low in saturated fat and cholesterol, may reduce the risk of heart disease.") A new study at Wake Forest University Baptist Medical Center in North Carolina found that a daily soy beverage containing 37 mg of isoflavones (the amount in 1 1/2 cups of soy milk) lowered high cholesterol by 8 percent. A daily drink with 62 mg of isoflavones decreased cholesterol 9 percent, but a drink with 27 mg of isoflavones had no benefit.

The higher your cholesterol, the greater the impact. A recent review of 38 studies in the *New England Journal of Medicine* showed that soy protein (average 47 grams daily) depressed high cholesterol (above 335) by 24 percent, compared with 8 percent when cholesterol was 200 or less. Soy worked regardless of levels of dietary fat.

Isoflavones and Cancer

Isoflavones are one of the five chemical classes of anticarcinogens found in soy. The others are as follows:

Phytate. In test-tube experiments, it inhibited the growth of human leukemia, colon and prostate cancer cells. It is also involved in regulating vital cellular functions such as signal transduction, cell proliferation and cell differentiation.

Phytosterol. Phytosterols are also believed to reduce cholesterol levels by inhibiting cholesterol absorption thus reducing the risk of heart disease.

Protease inhibitors. These protect against the damaging effects of radiation and free radicals, which can attack DNA.

Saponins. Saponins are a large family of modified carbohydrates found in many vegetables and herbs. So far, researchers have identified eleven different saponins in soybeans alone. In addition to being anticarcinogens, there is evidence that some of these substances lower circulating levels of certain lipids.

Studies show isoflavones can slow prostate cancer cells from growing, according to a study published in the June 2000 issue of the *International Journal of Oncology*. In 2001, researchers at Harvard Medical School presented their findings from a new study showing that mice inoculated with cancer cells had their tumors sharply reduced with a soy diet. After eight weeks, tumor size was reduced by 68 percent, and the spread of tumors to lymph nodes reduced by 50 percent in the soy-treated mice, compared to the untreated group.

In a recent study that tracked 12,395 Seventh-day Adventist men found that those who drank soy milk more than once a day were 70 percent less likely to get prostate cancer.

Estrogen promotes cancers of the prostate, breast, ovaries, and endometrium, and soy may diminish estrogen's activity. The phytoestrogens in soy have a structure similar to that of regular estrogen, so the soy phytoestrogens bind to the estrogen receptors but do not turn these receptors on to the same degree as regular estrogen. Once the soy phytoestrogens bind to these receptors, they keep regular estrogen from binding to it, thereby lessening estrogen's effects.

It's believed isoflavones can prevent the growth of estrogen-dependent breast cancer cells, according to findings published in the March 2000 issue of *Cancer Research*. That's because isoflavones appear to encourage the body to break down estrogen more quickly before it can stimulate cancer cells to grow. Instead of lingering in the blood, bits and pieces of estrogen molecules wind up in the urine.

Here's the Flip Side

Soy supplements are widely promoted as a "natural" way to reduce menopausal symptoms such as hot flashes, and for other proposed health benefits, especially for women who don't want to eat soy foods regularly. Isoflavones are found in soy, certain herbs, grains, and seeds, notably flaxseed. These are supposed to replenish the aging body's declining estrogen levels and thus relieve menopausal symptoms, as well as decrease the risk of heart disease and osteoporosis, without promoting breast cancer. At least that's the theory. Two of the primary soy isoflavones, genistein and daidzein, are found in many supplements. These may indeed affect the risk of cancer, especially breast cancer—but for better or worse?

Almost all of the research on isolated isoflavones has been done on animals or in the test tube and no one knows for certain how these animal and test tube studies relate to humans.

Some animal studies suggest that these substances may help maintain bone strength and inhibit certain cancers. Other studies suggest that it isn't the genistein and daidzein— or any of the other isoflavones or isoflavone compounds—but something else in soy that provides these benefits. Plus, there have been other studies into various proposed health benefits of soy or soy compounds that have not found a positive effect. Some research has found that the isoflavones may inhibit thyroid function.

Also, while the phytoestrogens and isoflavones bind to the estrogen receptors and only weakly stimulate these receptors and keep regular estrogen from more strongly turning them on, too much of even the weakly stimulating phytoestrogens and isoflavones may be unwise. One study showing that women who took purified isoflavones in pill or powder form consumed excessive amounts of these and thus increased their risk of breast cancer. If you have breast cancer, it's probably a good idea to eat soy but to avoid purified isoflavone supplements, keeping under 25–50 mg of isoflavones per day.

Obviously, not everyone is climbing on the soy bandwagon. Some researchers now worry that too much of a good thing could be harmful. Lon White, M.D., M.P.H., senior neuroepidemiologist at the University of Hawaii, is concerned soy may speed the aging of brain cells. He recently found evidence that the brains of elderly people who ate tofu at least twice a week for thirty years were aging faster than normal. Tests designed to assess memory and analytical ability showed that their brains functioned as if they were four years older than their actual age, White says of his study published in the April 2000 issue of the *Journal of the American College of Nutrition*.

Another fear is that the estrogen-like substances in soy may dampen the function of the thyroid. Consuming 40 mg of isoflavones a day can slow the production of thyroid hormone, said Dr. Gillespie. (One tablespoon of soy powder contains about 25 mg of isoflavones, and most isoflavone supplements come in 40 mg pills.)

According to Dr. Gillespie, within a few weeks of regularly consuming 40 mg of isoflavones, some women feel fatigued, constipated and achy all over. Some also gain weight and have heavier menstrual periods. Menopausal women are at particular risk, since they're already prone to hypothyroidism. "Women think it's because of hormones and don't realize they're symptoms of hypothyroidism," Gillespie says. "Once they stop the soy, they say, 'I'm feeling fine again.'"

Although studies point to dangers from soy, others suggest important benefits. On balance, soy, so far, has proven to be a superb food for people with prostate cancer and for those trying to prevent it.

How to Add Soy to Your Diet

On balance, soy appears to be a safe, and effective food, if eaten in moderation. (Two or three times per week.) Although soy foods are well worth adding to your diet, supplements containing concentrated isoflavones are another matter. No one knows what the long-term effects are. (By "soy supplements" I mean capsules and pills, not soy powders or soy concentrates, which contain relatively low levels of isoflavones per serving.)

Proponents and marketers of the supplements don't mention all the unknowns and the possible adverse effects. If isolated isoflavones have unpredictable hormonal actions in the body; that's risky business. Pregnant or nursing women, in particular, shouldn't risk taking isoflavone supplements. In contrast, people have been eating soy foods for centuries, and there's good evidence that these are healthful.

For now, at least, there is no major pill to gain the benefits from all known phytochemicals. Researchers continue to investigate the interactions of phytochemicals naturally present in food, but the relationship between them is very complicated and the picture is not anywhere near complete.

But even if some day we can buy them, they will most likely only provide selected components in a concentrated form, not the diversity of compounds that occur naturally in foods. So, it is important to stress increased fruit, vegetable, and grain consumption to acquire the benefits of phytochemicals than holding out hope for a magic pill containing these substances. Are there any negative effects?

Individual phytochemicals have been and continue to be evaluated for their safety and effectiveness in regard to disease prevention. Although most studies are positive, there are a few studies involving animals that show possible detrimental effects. These studies involve animals and specific phytochemicals in high dosages. However, the safety of consuming large amounts of fruits, vegetables and grains is not presently a concern.

Despite all the good news, it's important to also offer a word of warning. Like any other "newly" discovered chemical, there is a need for further investigation for potential health benefits and possible health risks. Optimal levels of individual phytochemicals have yet to be resolved and full understanding of requirements during various states of disease might differ from requirements for prevention of the same diseases. At this time, researchers just don't know how much people should add to their diets, especially when you factor in requirements for different genders, age groups, body types, and so forth that also need further study. The best bet is to not experiment with supplements, but not worry in the least about packing away as many fruits and vegetables as possible.

I'm Sold on Antioxidants—What Next?

First, it is important for Americans to become aware of their lack of consumption of fruits, vegetables and grains. Numerous studies by major health organizations show the average American consumes only one serving of vegetables and one serving of fruit each day. In one 1996 survey published in the *Journal of the American Dental Association*, one in every nine Americans ate no fruit or vegetable on the day they were interviewed.

Increasing the consumption of plant products in one's diet should not be difficult or time consuming. There are plenty of simple strategies for increasing dietary fruits, vegetables, and grains, including the suggestions below:

- Reach for juice instead of coffee or soda.
- Add chopped fruit to cereal, yogurt, pancakes, muffins, or even a milkshake.
- Snack on fresh chopped carrots, celery, broccoli, cauliflower, peppers and other vegetables.

- Add fresh greens, carrots, celery, parsley, tomatoes, and/or beans to your soups.
- Store dried fruit (apricots, dates, raisins, and more) for a quick snack at home or work.
- Eat soy a couple of times per week.
- Keep fruits and vegetables stocked and in sight. Fresh is best but frozen and canned (without syrup) will do.

It's long been believed that processed fruits and vegetables have a lower nutritional value than fresh produce. Not so, say Cornell University researchers. In a recent study, they found cooked sweet corn, for example, retains its antioxidant activity despite the loss of some vitamin C.

In their study, the researchers purchased sweet corn and cooked the kernels in batches at 115 degrees Celsius for ten, twenty-five, and fifty minutes. The cooking increased the antioxidant in sweet corn by 22, 44, and 53 percent respectively, said Liu Ruihai, Cornell assistant professor of food science. Reporting in the August 14, 2002 issue of *Journal of Agriculture and Food Chemistry*, they found that in addition to its antioxidant benefits, cooked sweet corn unleashes a phenolic compound called ferulic acid, which has added health benefits, such as battling cancer. Ferulic acid is a compound related to vanillin and is obtained from certain plants.

Obviously, the effects of antioxidants are crucial to our health, and I've covered a lot of different nutrients and chemical substances in these last two chapters. Believe it or not, there are even more antioxidants I haven't covered that are generating a fair share of publicity. I'll cover these in the next chapter.

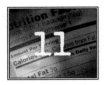

Even More Antioxidants

The previous two chapters covered many of the food components that can help thwart the ravage of free radicals. There are other very important substances that also act as antioxidants. Here are a few of the best known and most publicized.

Ginkgo Biloba

For centuries, extracts from the leaves of the *Ginkgo biloba* tree have been used as Chinese herbal medicine to treat a variety of medical conditions. In Europe and some Asian countries, standardized extracts from ginkgo leaves are taken to treat a wide range of symptoms, including dizziness, memory impairment, inflammation, and reduced blood flow to the brain and other areas of impaired circulation. Because *Ginkgo biloba* is an antioxidant, some claims have been made that it can be used to prevent damage caused by free radicals.

Ginkgo contains antioxidant flavonoids including ginkgo flavones or glycosides, and terpenoids such as ginkgolides and bilabolide. In the U.S., ginkgo is used to treat symptoms connected with decreased blood flow to the brain, particularly in elderly people. These symptoms include short-term memory loss and dizziness. Other symptoms ginkgo can treat include ringing in the ears, headache, depression, erectile dysfunction and anxiety. Circulation problems in the legs also have responded to ginkgo.

Ginkgo has been the focus of recent media reports as a potential treatment for Alzheimer's disease. Researchers at the New York Institute for Medical Research in Tarrytown, New York, conducted the first clinical study of *Ginkgo biloba* and dementia in the United States. Their findings were published in the *Journal of the American Medical Association* in October 1997.

These scientists examined how taking 120 mg a day of a *Ginkgo biloba* extract affected the rate of cognitive decline in people with mild to moderately severe dementia due to Alzheimer's disease and vascular dementia. Three tests were used to measure changes in the condition of participants.

First, participants showed a slight improvement on a test that measured their cognitive function (mental processes of knowing, thinking, and learning). Second, participants showed a slight improvement on a test that measured social behavior and mood changes that were observed by their caregivers. Third, participants showed no improvement on a doctor's assessment of change test.

Because 60 percent of the people did not complete the study, findings are difficult to interpret and may even be distorted. In addition, this study did not address the effect of *Ginkgo biloba* on delaying or preventing the onset of Alzheimer's disease or vascular dementia. The researchers recommend more investigation to determine if these findings are valid, understand how *Ginkgo biloba* works on brain cells, and identify an effective dosage and potential side effects. At the end of the study, they reported ginkgo might be of some help in treating the symptoms of Alzheimer's disease and vascular dementia, but there was no evidence that *Ginkgo biloba* will cure or prevent Alzheimer's disease.

Other studies also show ginkgo provides modest benefit for people with established dementia. Not only has any benefit been shown taking gingko as a preventive measure to avoid the development of Alzheimer's or dementia, there is scant evidence that gingko enhances normal memory. In fact, the results of a six-week study published in the August 21, 2002, issue of the *Journal of the American Medical Association* indicate that ginkgo does not improve learning, memory, attention and concentration in elderly adults with normal cognitive function. More studies are needed, however, on the effect of long-term use.

Although Germany recently approved ginkgo extracts (240 mg a day) to treat Alzheimer's disease, there is not enough information to recommend its broad use. Much more research is needed before scientists will know whether and how *Ginkgo biloba* extracts benefit people.

In Europe, doctors commonly prescribe *Ginkgo biloba* supplements to patients who have peripheral artery disease—a narrowing of arteries due to cholesterol buildup. Here in the United States, *Ginkgo biloba* supplements are among the most popular on the market with consumers spending upward of $240 million on the herbal products in 1997 alone. But whether it really helps treat peripheral artery disease remains an open question.

Ginkgo precautions. Possible side affects from taking ginkgo include muscle spasms, allergic skin reactions, cramps, bleeding, and mild digestive problems. Don't use ginkgo it if you're taking anticlotting medication including a regular dose aspirin. Also avoid using it if you're taking a thiazide diuretic. Ginkgo may raise blood pressure if used with this drug. Don't take it if you're pregnant. Discontinue taking gingko at least seven days prior to surgery.

Ginseng

Panax ginseng (Asian, Korean, and Chinese) is best known for its ability to help the body deal with stress by allowing for a more consistent energy level. It now appears that the health benefits of ginseng go beyond stress reduction. Researchers are learning that this herb might help fight diabetes, heart disease and cancer.

An integral part of Chinese medicine for more than two thousand years, ginseng root is known as an "adaptogenic" herb. That is, it increases the body's resistance to stress and balances functions of the immune, nervous and cardiovascular systems. The active ingredients in the herb help reduce stress by stimulating the adrenal glands. These triangular-shaped glands sit above your kidneys and regulate the release of stress hormones. With chronic fatigue or stress, adrenal function can become compromised, affecting the body's release of hormones and immune compounds as well as diminishing the overall feeling of energy.

In the Orient, ginseng is used to treat diabetes. Animal studies have shown that the herb enhances the release of insulin from the pancreas and increases the body's sensitivity to insulin. In doing so, ginseng allows the maintenance of more stable blood sugar levels.

A Finnish study investigated the effect of 100 mg and 200 mg of *Panax ginseng* on blood sugar control in thirty-six people with type II (non-insulin dependent) diabetes. After eight weeks, both doses of ginseng elevated mood and reduced fasting blood sugar.

Ginseng for Your Heart

A number of animal studies have shown the ability of ginseng to lower elevated levels of blood cholesterol. It appears that ginseng compounds inhibit the production of cholesterol in the liver. As an antioxidant, ginseng may protect artery walls and LDL (bad) cholesterol from oxidative damage caused by harmful free radical molecules. Once LDL cholesterol is oxidized, it readily sticks to artery walls.

Ginseng's antioxidant action also has the potential to protect us from cancer. In fact, a recent study found that ginseng, together with vitamins E, C and beta-carotene, decreased the amount of oxidized molecules in the blood of smokers.

Ginseng also has immune-enhancing properties. A large Italian study found that individuals taking 100 mg of standardized ginseng (G115 extract) produced significantly higher levels of antibodies in response to a flu shot compared to those who did not take the herb. Killer white blood cells were nearly twice as high in the ginseng group after eight weeks of supplementation. These and other white blood cells are an important part of the body's defense against viruses and foreign molecules.

Ginseng and Concentration

It's long been thought that ginseng enhances concentration and sharpens thinking. A recent Danish study investigated the effects of 400 mg of *Panax ginseng* on 112 healthy middle-aged adults. After eight weeks, those who took ginseng had greater abstract thinking ability and significantly improved reaction time to auditory prompts. No significant differences were noted in memory or concentration.

Researchers have also shown that the active ingredients in the herb can increase oxygen uptake by muscles, avoiding the fatigue caused by oxygen deprivation. European studies found that oxygen transportation to body tissues was increased by as much as 29 percent. Other studies have found similar results in athletes.

How to Take Ginseng

Many of ginseng's health benefits can be attributed to active compounds, in the root called ginsenosides. Many ginsenosides, have been identified in ginseng root, but Rg1 and Rb1 have received the most attention. Scientific research has focused mainly on ginseng extracts standardized to contain four to seven per cent ginsenosides.

To purchase a high-quality product, look for a statement of standardization or "G115" on the label. The usual dosage of a standardized extract is 100 or 200 mg, once daily. If you are using the dried root, take one to two grams a day in the form of tea or capsules. Take ginseng for two to three weeks and follow with a one to two week rest period.

Ginseng is relatively safe at the 100 or 200 mg dosage. In some people, it may cause mild stomach upset, irritability and insomnia. To avoid overstimulation start with 100 mg a day and avoid taking the herb with caffeine. Ginseng should not be used during pregnancy, breastfeeding, or in individuals with uncontrolled high blood pressure.

Unlike Panax or Asian ginseng, Siberian ginseng has a milder effect and pregnant and nursing women can safely take Siberian ginseng. It is also much less likely to cause over-stimulation in sensitive individuals. Choose a product standardized for eleutherosides B and E. The usual dosage is 300 to 400 mg once daily for six to eight weeks, followed by a one to two week break. Products labeled as American ginseng are not really a ginseng at all.

Ginseng helps the body deal with life's daily stresses and provides long-term adrenal support. In conjunction with a plant-based diet, regular exercise and antioxidant supplements like vitamin E and ginkgo, ginseng just might help you live healthier.

Melatonin

This antioxidant hormone produced by the brain's pineal gland during sleep has been touted as a natural way to get a better night's sleep, to improve one's sex life, to live longer and to fight the ravages of AIDS, Alzheimer's disease and cancer, among other afflictions. Melatonin production normally peaks around the time of puberty and then decreases with age.

Although some people claim it helps them with all of the above, there's a great amount of research that doesn't support these wonderful claims. In fact, a backlash against melatonin hype is now under way. Critics warn that the doses of melatonin commonly sold in health food stores that raise levels of the substance in the blood thirty-fold higher than their normal peak, could be dangerous for some people. And many researchers point out that the more startling claims being made for the substance are unsupported by studies on patients, but rather extrapolations from experiments conducted on rats and mice. These animals differ from people in many ways, especially as regards sleep, the one aspect of human physiology that melatonin clearly affects.

In about 10 percent of the people followed thus far in studies of the hormone, high doses of melatonin have caused insomnia and nightmares rather than peaceful sleep. One high-dose study noted mental impairment in subjects, and subjects in another study reported severe headaches. Very high doses of melatonin have been found to affect other hormones. Estrogen, testosterone and thyroid hormone production are decreased by high-dose melatonin. Melatonin also may affect the immune system. The hormone may be viewed as giving immunity a "boost," but this is not necessarily a positive effect for some people, including those with autoimmune disorders.

Although melatonin can affect some reproductive hormones, it has never been demonstrated to enhance sexual performance in humans. Indeed, Dr. William Regelson, coauthor of the book *The Melatonin Miracle*, admitted in a television appearance that the claim on his book cover that melatonin is a sex enhancer is simply a promotional claim, not a scientifically demonstrated fact.

Richard Wurtman, a researcher at the Massachusetts Institute of Technology, has spent years studying melatonin and its biological effects. He has described some of that work in a January 1989 Scientific American article entitled "Carbohydrates and Depression." Wurtman says there is no doubt that the substance, in doses of a fraction of a milligram, can induce sleep and shift the sleep cycle.

But Wurtman, who holds an M.I.T. patent covering the use of melatonin for controlling sleep, says there is no evidence that it has any effect on human life expectancy, and "only marginal" evidence that it promotes longevity in mice.

Wurtman further argues health-food store doses of melatonin might diminish sex drive. He also denounces as "wicked" the suggestion that people with cancer or AIDS should take the hormone. Wurtman thinks melatonin is as likely to worsen those conditions as to ease them.

Wurtman is not the only researcher criticizing melatonin mania. In a 2001 article published in the journal *Cell*, Steven M. Reppert and David R. Weaver of Harvard Medical School described as "seriously flawed" an experiment by Walter Pierpaoli, William Regelson and others that raised hopes melatonin might extend life.

The investigators prolonged the life of elderly mice by giving them transplants of tissue from the pineal gland taken from younger mice. Pierpaoli and Regelson, authors of the book, *The Melatonin Miracle*, hypothesized that the transplanted tissue was more responsive to melatonin and somehow revitalized the old mice. But according to Reppert and Weaver, the mice used in the experiments have a genetic defect that means they cannot make melatonin; discrediting their assertion of the hormone's miraculous effect.

Fred W. Turek of Northwestern University, writing in *Nature*, points out that "not one study" in humans supports Pierpaoli and Regelson's claim that, for example, melatonin helps to prevent heart attacks. Victor Herbert and Ruth Cava of the American Council on Science and Health caution that children, women who are nursing or who may become pregnant, and people who have immune-system disorders should avoid taking the hormone because of uncertainties about its effects.

Melatonin strategies. Anyone suffering from occasional insomnia who is interested in taking melatonin to deal with this condition should make sure:

- the dosage is not above the effective level; i.e., 0.1–0.3 mg
- he or she takes it at the appropriate time; i.e., in the evening, about one half hour before going to bed
- he or she takes it under appropriate medical supervision

As you might be aware, sleep-promoting compounds are found in a number of foods. Rather than popping a pill at bedtime, a person with a mild case of sleeplessness could try a bedtime snack that includes foods such as milk, peanuts, turkey, chicken or almonds. All of these foods contain tryptophan, which raises brain serotonin that in turn can be converted to melatonin.

Superoxide Dismutase (SOD)

Superoxide dismutase (SOD), an extremely potent antioxidant enzyme, fights cellular damage from free radicals and helps keep our cell membranes young, supple and healthy. SOD helps the body utilize zinc, copper and manganese; and SOD injections have been shown to help treat scleroderma, a hardening of the skin. The best natural sources of SOD are barley grass, broccoli, Brussels sprouts, cabbage and wheatgrass.

This enzyme converts oxygen radicals, which are normal by-products of cell metabolism, to hydrogen peroxide and water. Glutathione peroxidase then converts the hydrogen peroxide to water and oxygen.

One theory states that if there is more SOD without a corresponding increase in glutathione peroxidase, then more hydrogen peroxide becomes available to cause damage to the cell. Experiments with cell cultures and postmortem tests seem to show that this oxidative damage might cause premature aging, damage leading to senile dementia including Alzheimer's, and the early loss of brain cells seen in infants with Down syndrome. However, no evidence of this oxidative damage has been found in living humans with Down syndrome.

I've spent a great deal of time on antioxidants. But these vitamins, minerals and other compounds make up only part of the important nutrients we need. There are plenty of other vitamins and minerals available to us when we follow a sound eating plan—as you'll see in the next chapter.

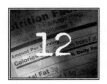

Our Real Needs for Other Vitamins

As I've already pointed out, nutritional research in the past focused on preventing vitamin deficiencies. Now, scientists are investigating specific vitamins for preventing and treating disease and for enhancing physical and mental health and performance. Despite exciting work in this area, it's still not the emphasis of our government's nutritional standards.

Beyond that, it's commonly accepted we need vitamins for normal body functions, mental alertness and resistance to infection. They enable our bodies to process proteins, carbohydrates and fats. Certain vitamins also help us produce blood cells, hormones, genetic material and chemicals in our nervous systems. Unlike carbohydrates, proteins and fats, vitamins and minerals don't provide fuel in the form of calories. However, they help our bodies release and use calories from food.

Vitamins are also key components of enzymes and coenzymes. Enzymes speed up chemical reactions in the body either by building or breaking chemical bonds that create molecules. Coenzymes help the enzymes in their chemical reactions.

As a reminder, vitamins are generally divided into two groups, water soluble and fat soluble. The water-soluble vitamins are very safe. They are readily excreted from the body and are not stored.

The fat-soluble vitamins are stored in the fat tissue and fatty organs like the liver. You can therefore experience toxicity from these vitamins if you take them in large quantities.

I've already talked about the antioxidant vitamins in a previous chapter. They are as follows:

- vitamin A (fat soluble; stored in body fat):
- vitamin E (fat soluble)
- vitamin C (water soluble)

There are other vitamins we need to know about. The first group of these is the fat-soluble vitamins. They are as follows:

- vitamin D
- vitamin K
- choline; part of the B complex. (No RDA/DRI established)

Water-soluble vitamins (stored in the body to a lesser extent than fat-soluble vitamins) are as follows:

- thiamin (B1)
- riboflavin (B2)
- niacin (B3)
- pantothenic acid (B5) (no RDA/DRI established)
- pyridoxine (B6)
- biotin (B7)
- folic acid/folate (B9)
- cobalamin (B12)
- inositol (no RDA/DRI established)
- PABA (para-aminobenzoic acid) (no RDA/DRI established)

For your convenience, I'll repeat the RDA/DRI charts from Chapter 2. Don't feel you have to study them, though; they can be very confusing.

Table 12.1 Comparisons of RDIs, DRIs, and ULs for Vitamins

VITAMIN	Current RDI*	New DRI†	UL‡
Vitamin A	5000 IU	3000 IU	10000 IU
Vitamin C	60 mg	90 mg	2000 mg
Vitamin D	10 mcg	15 mcg	50 mcg
Vitamin E	20 mg	15 mg	1000 mg
Vitamin K	80 mcg	120 mcg	ND
Thiamin	1.5 mg	1.2 mg	ND
Riboflavin	1.7 mg	1.3 mg	ND
Niacin	20 mg	16 mg	35 mg
Vitamin B6	2 mg	1.7 mg	100 mg
Folate	400 mcg	400 mcg	1000 mcg
Vitamin B12	6 mcg	2.4 mcg	ND
Biotin	300 mcg	30 mcg	ND
Pantothenic	10 mg	5 mg	ND
Choline	ND	550 mg	3500 mg

* The Reference Daily Intake (RDI) is the value established by the Food and Drug Administration (FDA) for use in nutrition labeling. It was based initially on the highest 1968 Recommended Dietary Allowance (RDA) for each nutrient, to assure that needs were met for all age groups.

† The Dietary Reference Intakes (DRI) are the most recent set of dietary recommendations established.

‡ The Upper Limit (UL) is the upper level of intake considered to be safe for use by adults, incorporating a safety factor. In some cases, lower ULs have been established for children.

ND Upper Limit not determined. No adverse effects observed from high intakes of the nutrient.

Charts are very useful, but they can't show you everything. Here's what you should know about the remaining vitamins.

Vitamin D (calciferol)

The major function of vitamin D is to maintain normal blood levels of calcium and phosphorus helping—along with a number of other vitamins, minerals, and hormones—to form and maintain strong bones and teeth. Without vitamin D, bones can become thin, brittle, soft or misshapen. Vitamin D prevents rickets in children and osteomalacia, or soft bones, in adults, which are skeletal diseases that result in defects that weaken bones.

Vitamin D is also referred to as the sunshine vitamin, since the body, in a sunny climate can manufacture this nutrient from sunshine on your skin using cholesterol from your body to do so. (It's important to remember that this can be achieved in about thirty minutes by fair skinned people, while dark skinned people, because of the pigmentation need about three hours to reach the same level of manufacture.)

'Dem Bones

Researchers know that normal bone is constantly being broken down and rebuilt even in adults—maybe that should be ESPECIALLY in adults. In adults with prolonged vitamin D deficiency, the collagenous bone matrix is preserved but bone mineral is progressively lost as a result of normal bone "turnover," resulting in bone pain and soft bones known as osteomalacia.

Although they both result in fragile bones, osteomalacia differs from osteoporosis in several ways. Osteomalacia is relatively rare and characterized by decreased bone mineral content in the presence of a relative increase in the bone matrix. In contrast, osteoporosis is characterized by a decrease in total bone mass, with no change in the ratio of bone mineral to the bone matrix.

It is estimated that over twenty-five million adults in the United States have, or are at risk of developing osteoporosis, a disease characterized by fragile bones resulting in an increased risk of bone fractures. Having normal storage levels of vitamin D in your body helps keep your bones strong and can help prevent osteoporosis in elderly individuals, in post-menopausal women and in individuals on chronic steroid therapy.

During menopause, the balance between the building up and tearing down of our bones is upset, resulting in more bone being broken down or reabsorbed than rebuilt.

Vitamin D and the Heart

Proper levels of vitamin D might also lower the risk of death from heart disease by one-third, at least for women, according to research at the University of California, San Francisco (UCSF). In

April 2002, Dr. Paul D. Varosy told attendees of the 42nd annual conference on Cardiovascular Disease and Epidemiology Prevention in Honolulu, Hawaii that low levels of vitamin D in the blood have previously been linked with higher risk of heart disease and heart attacks. The researchers set out to determine if taking vitamin D supplements decreased this risk.

Dr. Varosy's team analyzed data from nearly ten thousand women over the age of sixty-five who were enrolled in a study of how often osteoporosis causes broken bones. Of these, more than 4,200 women reported that they took vitamin D supplements at the time of the study, and another 733 reported a prior history of supplement use.

After following the women for an average of nearly eleven years, Dr. Varosy and colleagues found that the risk of heart disease death was 31 percent lower in those women who were taking vitamin D at the time of the study.

The researchers note that calcium supplements, education, self-reported health status or health-related behaviors had no effect on the protection afforded by vitamin D. Dr. Varosy said it was important to note that the American Heart Association does not advocate the use of supplements, and he doesn't either. "They recommend getting adequate nutrients from food sources," said Dr. Varosy. "I still think that is the best way to go. This doesn't mean you should go out and start taking supplements. People should talk to their doctors first."

Here Comes the Sun

As I said earlier, we get vitamin D from dietary sources, but it can also generate on its own when sunlight converts a chemical in your skin into a usable form of the vitamin. Ultraviolet (UV) rays from sunlight trigger vitamin D synthesis in the skin. Season, latitude, time of day, cloud cover, smog and suncreens affect UV ray exposure. For example, in Boston the average amount of sunlight is insufficient to produce significant vitamin D synthesis in the skin from November through February.

Sunscreens with a sun protection factor of 8 or greater will block UV rays that produce vitamin D, but it is still important to routinely use sunscreen whenever sun exposure is longer than ten to fifteen minutes. It is especially important for individuals with limited sun exposure to include good sources of vitamin D in their diet.

Vitamin D and Cancer

Laboratory, animal and clinical studies suggest that vitamin D might offer protection from some cancers. Some dietary surveys have associated increased intake of dairy foods with decreased incidence of colon and breast cancer.

For example, studies at the Weill Medical College of Cornell University and The Rockefeller University in New York, found low levels of dietary calcium and vitamin D in a high-fat diet caused adverse changes in the mammary gland and several other organs. These risks were reversed by increasing dietary calcium and vitamin D. According to the researchers, the findings further suggest a possible role for increased dietary calcium and vitamin D in the prevention of these cancers. At the University of North Carolina, Chapel Hill, researchers found lower rates of prostate cancer in southern climates where there is more sunlight.

Researchers exploring the vitamin D/cancer connection say well-designed clinical trials need to be conducted to determine whether vitamin D deficiency increases cancer risk or whether an increased intake of vitamin D is protective against some cancers. Until such trials are conducted, it is premature to advise anyone to take vitamin D supplements to prevent cancer.

Vitamin D and Steroids

Corticosteroid medications are often prescribed to reduce inflammation from a variety of medical problems. These medicines may be essential for a person's medical treatment, but they have potential side effects, including decreased calcium absorption. There is some evidence that steroids may also impair vitamin D metabolism, further contributing to the loss of bone and development of osteoporosis associated with steroid medications.

Food sources. Vitamin D is found naturally in very few foods. Foods containing vitamin D include some fatty fish (herring, salmon, sardines), fish liver oils and eggs from hens that have been fed vitamin D. In the U.S., milk and infant formula are fortified with vitamin D to contain 10 mcg (400 IU)/quart. However, other dairy products such as cheese and yogurt are not usually fortified with vitamin D. Some cereals and breads are also fortified with vitamin D. Accurate estimates of average dietary intakes of vitamin D are difficult because of the high variability of the vitamin D content of fortified foods. As you probably know, dairy products as sources of calcium and vitamin D are controversial. I'll offer both sides of the argument in the next chapter.

Supplemental advice. If you don't consume dietary sources of calcium, have dark skin, are at risk of osteoporosis, live in a cloudy environment or rarely go outside, or take certain medications, you might consider taking a vitamin D supplement to meet your daily requirement. Studies show that people who supplement their diets with a combination of vitamin D and calcium slow their bone loss and reduce their number of fractures. But don't do it on your own. Consult with your doctor first.

A greater vitamin D intake from diet and supplements has been associated with less bone loss in older women. Since bone loss increases the risk of fractures, vitamin D supplementation may help prevent fractures resulting from osteoporosis.

Treatment of vitamin D deficiency can result in decreased incidence of hip fractures, and daily supplementation with 20 mcg (800 IU) of vitamin D may reduce the risk of osteoporotic fractures in elderly populations with low blood levels of vitamin D.

See your doctor before taking vitamin D if you have epilepsy, heart or blood vessel disease, chronic diarrhea, disease of the kidney, liver or pancreas, intestinal problems, sarcoidosis (an immune system disorder) or if you're planning to become pregnant. If you're pregnant or breast-feeding, don't take vitamin D in doses greater than the RDA for pregnant or breast-feeding women.

Symptoms of deficiency. Vitamin D deficiency, which occurs more often in post-menopausal women and older Americans, has been associated with greater incidence of hip fractures. In one study, a group of women with osteoporosis hospitalized for hip fractures, 50 percent were found to have signs of vitamin D deficiency.

Symptoms of toxicity. Vitamin D toxicity is also called, hypervitaminosis D. Hypervitaminosis D appears to result primarily from vitamin D supplementation over many years at doses of 10,000 to

50,000 IU/day (250 to 1250 mcg/day). Symptoms include loss of appetite, nausea, vomiting, excessive thirst, excessive urination, severe itching, muscular weakness, joint pain, and ultimately disorientation, coma and death. Also, blood and urinary calcium levels are elevated. If the condition persists, demineralization of bones and deposits of calcium in soft tissues, such as the heart and kidneys, can also occur. No cases of vitamin D toxicity have been observed from sun exposure.

Vitamin K

Vitamin K is essential for the functioning of several proteins involved in blood clotting. In fact, vitamin K's "K" designation is derived from the German word "koagulation."

Vitamin K can be acquired by our bodies from several sources:

- vitamin K1 or phylloquinone is from plants
- vitamin K2, menaquinone is made by intestinal bacteria
- vitamin K3 is manufactured synthetically

Besides blood clotting, vitamin K might also be useful in osteoporosis, cancer prevention and heart disease. Although vitamin K is a fat-soluble vitamin, the body stores very little of it, and its stores are rapidly depleted without regular amounts added from the diet. Perhaps, because of its limited ability to store vitamin K, the body recycles it through a process called "the vitamin K cycle."

It is given to some patients before surgery to prevent excessive bleeding after the operation. Other uses of vitamin K are to build strong bones by helping the body use calcium and to slow excessive menstrual bleeding. Vitamin K can be used topically to help the skin heal from wounds, including surgical incisions, burns, bruises, scars and stretch marks. Supplements of vitamin K generally are not necessary unless there is an intestinal problem with poor absorption.

Blood Clotting Problems

Some people are at risk of forming clots, which could block the flow of blood in arteries of the heart, brain or lungs, resulting in heart attack, stroke or pulmonary embolism. Some oral anticoagulants, such as warfarin (also known as coumarin or coumadin) aspirin as well as certain antibiotics inhibit the coagulation affect of vitamin K.

Vitamin K and Newborn Babies

Newborns are given one vitamin K1 injection soon after birth to help prevent bleeding problems since they don't yet have bacteria in the gut to make vitamin K.

Newborn babies that are exclusively breast-fed are at increased risk of vitamin K deficiency for the following reasons:

1. Human milk is relatively low in vitamin K compared to formula.
2. The newborn's intestines are not yet colonized with bacteria that synthesize menaquinones.
3. The vitamin K cycle may not be fully functional in newborns, especially premature infants.

Infants whose mothers are on anticonvulsant medication to prevent seizures are also at risk of vitamin K deficiency. Vitamin K deficiency in newborns may result in a bleeding disorder called hemorrhagic disease of the newborn (HDN). Because HDN is life threatening and easily prevented, the American Academy of Pediatrics and a number of similar international organizations recommend that an injection of phylloquinone (vitamin K1) be administered to all newborns.

Controversy arose regarding the routine use of vitamin K injections for newborns in the early 1990s when two retrospective studies were published suggesting the possibility of an association between vitamin K injections in newborns and the development of childhood leukemia and other forms of childhood cancer. However, two other large retrospective studies in the U.S. and Sweden that reviewed the medical records of 54,000 and 1.3 million children, respectively, found no evidence of a relationship between childhood cancers and vitamin K injections at birth. In a policy statement, the American Academy of Pediatrics recommended that routine vitamin K prophylaxis for newborns be continued because HDN is life-threatening and the risks of cancer are unproven and unlikely.

Only a handful of researchers worldwide study vitamin K. But with the aging of the U.S. population, this vitamin could command a bigger following as its role in the integrity of bones becomes increasingly clear. According to Sarah Booth of the Vitamin K Laboratory at the Jean Mayer USDA Human Nutrition Research Center on Aging at Tufts University in Boston, vitamin K activates at least three proteins involved in bone health. Booth said while in the past it looked like Americans consumed several times the recommended dietary allowance for vitamin K, improved analytical methods show that the vitamin isn't as abundant in the diet as once thought.

In a recent survey, after studying the estimated vitamin K intake from self-reported fourteen-day food intake diaries of two thousand households across the U.S., she and her research team found people between the ages of eighteen and forty-four weren't getting enough vitamin K. Phylloquinone, the most common form of vitamin K, was the researchers' benchmark for vitamin K intake.

"People over age sixty-five consumed more phylloquinone than those in the twenty to forty age bracket," said Booth. "Only half the females age thirteen and over and less than half the males got the RDA. This confirms there are very low intakes nationwide."

Phylloquinone is found in some oils, especially soybean oil and in dark-green vegetables such as spinach and broccoli. One serving of spinach or two servings of broccoli provide four to five times the RDA of phylloquinone.

Booth said recent evidence suggests the current RDA might not be sufficient for maximizing vitamin K's function in bones. The vitamin adds chemicals called carboxyl groups to osteocalcin and other proteins that build and maintain bone. Exactly how much vitamin K is needed to do this is unknown.

Most of the survey respondents also consumed another form of vitamin K (dihydrophylloquinone) produced during the hydrogenation of oils. About half of U.S. soybean oil is hydrogenated, according to the Institute of Shortening and Edible Oils in Washington, D.C. The degree of hydrogenation ranges from light, for margarines, spreads and cooking oils used in restaurants, to heavy, for deep frying and bakery products.

Booth said as much as 30 percent of total vitamin K intake can come from dihydrophylloquinone, which is less biologically active than phylloquinone. In fact, in the study it was found to be half as active with a clot-forming protein and was completely inactive with a bone-forming protein. "So hydrogenated oils shouldn't be considered an important source of vitamin K," said Booth.

Food sources. Phylloquinone (vitamin K1) is the major dietary form of vitamin K. Green leafy vegetables including spinach, green cabbage, kale, Swiss chard and turnip greens are richest in vitamin K. Broccoli, tomatoes, liver and lean meats and dairy products, are other good sources. Some vegetable oils (soybean, cottonseed, canola and olive) are major contributors of dietary vitamin K.

Supplemental advice. Since it is made by bacteria in the intestines, the need for supplements is low unless there is a problem with absorption.

Side effects. Very few side effects have been reported from the oral use of vitamin K. Some stomach irritation has been seen and in rare cases, usually in newborns, hemolytic anemia and thrombocytopenia.

Symptoms of deficiency. Vitamin K deficiency is uncommon in healthy adults. In fact, a deficiency is rarely seen unless there is an intestinal problem with fat absorption such as is seen in sprue, inflammatory bowel disease, liver disease, bowel obstruction or in people on long-term antibiotics. (Sprue, also known as Celiac disease, is a digestive disease that damages the small intestine and interferes with absorption of nutrients from food.)

Vitamin K deficiency results in impaired blood clotting. Symptoms include easy bruising and bleeding often appearing as nosebleeds, bleeding gums, blood in the urine, blood in the stool, tarry black stools or extremely heavy menstrual bleeding. A long-term deficiency of vitamin K can affect the bones, causing poor growth or osteoporosis.

Symptoms of toxicity. It is hard to get too much vitamin K as the body regulates the absorption. Large doses, however, may cause flushing and sweating. In some cases, hemolytic anemia, a condition in which the red blood cells die faster than usual and the body can't replace them quick enough, occurs. Too much vitamin K either from a change in diet or the addition of a supplement, will reverse the effects of oral anticoagulants such as warfarin.

Several drugs and vitamins can inhibit the effects of vitamin K and may cause bleeding. Vitamin E helps the body use vitamin K but too much vitamin E for a long time can inhibit vitamin K and cause bleeding. Vitamin A may also cause bleeding.

Taking aspirin over a long period of time may increase the need for vitamin K. Certain antibiotics, especially those called broad spectrum antibiotics, kill the vitamin K producing bacteria in the intestines and decrease the amount of vitamin K in the body, which may cause bleeding. Dilantin increases the metabolism of vitamin K, lowering the amount in the body and possibly causing bleeding.

The B-complex Vitamins

The vitamin B grouping or complex, refers to a selection of nutrients with some very similar properties, but are, in fact, separate nutrients. At first it was these similarities—and the fact that many of them are present in the same foods—that made researchers first think they were only parts of one vitamin. After closer examinations, it was found that there were several similar nutrients, which often work in synergy. Hence, the group was called the vitamin B complex, with each "part" receiving a separate designation, letter, descriptive name or chemical term.

Although I've included RDA/DRI charts for the B vitamins, I wouldn't put too much stock in them. Many scientists believe the DRIs for B vitamins should be higher. In 1995, a major study in the *New England Journal of Medicine* showed that people with high blood levels of the substance, homocysteine, were more likely to have clogged arteries, possibly leading to a heart attack. Three of the B vitamins—folic acid, pyridoxine, and cobalamin—break down homocysteine. The researchers found that the higher the levels of these three Bs, the lower the homocysteine level and the risk of heart attack.

Specifically, those with the highest B levels cut their risk of a heart attack in half. They also found two thirds of the people with dangerously high homocysteine had inadequate levels of the three vital Bs.

The Other B Vitamins

The following B vitamins don't have RDA/DRI values, even though all are important to our health:

* choline
* pantothenic acid (B5)

- inositol
- PABA (para-aminobenzoic acid)

Choline (no RDA/DRI established)

This B vitamin—which for some reason doesn't warrant a number—works closely with folic acid (B9) and cobalamin (B12) to make neurotransmitters, chemical messengers that carry information to and from your brain. It's also crucial for making the membranes of your cells.

Choline assists in controlling your weight as well as cholesterol levels, keeping cell membranes healthy and in preventing gallstones. It is also most useful in the maintenance of the nervous system, assisting memory and learning, and is believed to help fight infections, including hepatitis and AIDS. Choline is critical for normal membrane structure and function.

Choline is used by the kidneys to maintain water balance and also helps in critical liver functions. It is also used to produce the important neurotransmitter acetylcholine. It assists in nerve impulse transmission, gallbladder regulation, and lecithin production.

Should you consume alcohol, refined sugar or large amounts of nicotinic acid regularly, you might need extra choline. Choline, together with fat, inositol and essential unsaturated fatty acids, makes up lecithin, and needs a co-enzyme containing vitamin B6, and magnesium to be produced. If lecithin is in short supply it may allow your blood cholesterol levels to become elevated.

Food sources. Choline is found in egg yolks, beef, wheat germ, oats and nuts. Choline is lost in food processing, storage and cooking.

Supplemental advice. To use this vitamin therapeutically, the dosage is usually increased considerably, but the toxicity level must be kept in mind. The dosage is relative to the amount of fats ingested in the diet, but for a guide you can use male 550 mg/ per day and female 425 mg per day, although mega dose vitamin proponents use far higher dosages. The maximum level of choline has been set for safety at 3.5 g/day.

Choline should be taken in the same dose as inositol and together with the B group vitamins as well as vitamin A and linoleic acid.

Side effects. Taking too much choline could result in your body smelling fishy.

Symptoms of deficiency. A deficiency of choline does not happen easily but if it is deficient it may lead to liver disease, raised cholesterol levels, high blood pressure as well as kidney problems. Choline deficiency may also manifest itself in the inability to digest fats, stunted growth and fatty buildup in the liver. Memory and brain function could also be impaired.

Symptoms of toxicity. Too much choline can cause nausea, depression and could trigger existing epilepsy. Hypertension, sweating, salivation and diarrhea have also been reported.

Vitamin B1 (Thiamin)

Thiamin—also known as thiamine, or thiamin hydrochloride— prevents beriberi, a deficiency syndrome that affects the heart, gastrointestinal tract and nervous system.

Thiamin plays a role in many important reactions in the body and is needed with other B vitamins for energy production and the metabolism of carbohydrates. Vitamin B1 enhances circulation, helps with blood formation and is also needed by the nervous system for it to function properly. It helps improve mood, boost memory in dementia and Alzheimer's disease and prevent memory loss in the elderly. In children it is required for growth and has shown some indication to assist in arthritis, cataracts, as well as infertility.

It also helps to minimize numbness and tingling in the hands and feet as a result of diabetes. Thiamin has been used to treat depression, schizophrenia and the psychosis related to alcohol withdrawal. It also strengthens the heart, especially in congestive heart failure. It is also used in the manufacture of hydrochloric acid, and therefore plays a part in digestion.

Thiamin is very safe and there are no major side effects or toxicities associated with it. There are also few drug or supplement interactions.

Some foods have an effect on thiamin levels. Blueberries, red beet root, red cabbage, black currants, and Brussels sprouts decrease vitamin B1 levels. Drinking large quantities of tea and coffee, with or without caffeine, will also decrease levels. This is due to the tannins binding thiamin in the gut.

Drugs used for seizures, including Dilantin, can interfere with thiamin absorption and supplements may be necessary. Alcohol consumption, oral contraceptives and diuretics will also cause decreased thiamin stores.

Food sources. Thiamin is found in brewer's yeast, lean pork, wheat germ, sunflower seeds, pine nuts, soybeans and whole grain brown rice. Thiamin is destroyed by sulfites, a common food additive, and by moist heat and alkalis such as baking soda. Cooking also destroys thiamin in foods.

Supplemental advice. Very little of this vitamin is stored in the body, and depletion of this vitamin can happen within fourteen days.

Patients with dementia may be supplemented with up to 8 gm per day. Vitamin B1 should be taken with meals since the acid produced for digestion increases its absorption. If large amounts are taken daily, it is best to divide the dose and take a portion with each meal.

The requirement for thiamin increases as the caloric intake increases. Higher amounts are also needed in people eating high-carbohydrate diets or lots of junk food and those who have increased metabolism due to fever, exercise, overactive thyroid, pregnancy and stress.

Thiamin works closely with the other B vitamins and is best taken as a complex. The B vitamins should be taken in a one for one ratio. For example, a "B-complex 50" contains 50 mg of the vitamins B1, B2, B3, B6, choline, inositol and PABA, and 50 micrograms of vitamin B12, folic acid and biotin. Additional supplemental amounts of vitamin B1 can be added to this combination to suit individual needs.

Magnesium supplements may need to be taken with thiamin as magnesium is necessary to convert thiamin to its active form.

Side effects. Oral vitamin B1 rarely causes side effects but a hypersensitivity reaction can occur. More often, reactions occur to the injectable form and include tingling, pain, sweating, nausea, restlessness, difficulty breathing, a transient decrease in blood pressure and death.

Symptoms of deficiency. Symptoms of thiamin deficiency include tingling and numbness in the hands and feet, irritability, fatigue, weakness and muscle cramps in the legs, headache, insomnia, indigestion, weight loss, constipation, irregular heartbeat and high blood pressure. More severe symptoms include mental impairment, muscle wasting paralysis, nerve damage, and eventually death.

Symptoms of toxicity. The body eliminates this water-soluble vitamin so no toxicity has been seen.

Vitamin B2 (Riboflavin)

Riboflavin—also known as riboflavin-5-phosphate or flavin—is a very safe water-soluble vitamin. Physicians have used it to treat migraine headaches, cataracts and sickle-cell anemia. It has also been used for skin problems such as acne, seborrhea, athlete's foot, rosacea and cracks in the corners of the mouth. It may be useful for eye problems including blurred vision and eyes that are sensitive to light, eyes that tire easily and are bloodshot or watery.

Some problems with nerves or the nervous system, including nerve damage resulting in numbness and tingling, stress, tiredness, anxiety, depression, Alzheimer's disease and epilepsy have been treated with vitamin B2.

Riboflavin is also used to help the body detoxify environmental pollutants. It is needed for tissue repair and may be helpful in healing burns, injuries and wounds, including surgical incisions.

Vitamin B2 is also needed by the body to make red blood cells. It might also prevent the development of esophageal cancer.

Riboflavin is needed to make two enzymes, FMN (flavin mononucleotide) and FAD (flavin adenine dinucleotide) which are involved in energy metabolism. It helps regenerate glutathione, an antioxidant needed by the liver for the metabolism of drugs and environmental pollutants. Riboflavin also increases iron binding capacity and therefore the ability of the body to make red blood cells.

Psyllium (e.g. Metamucil), alcohol, oral contraceptives and some antibiotics slow the absorption of vitamin B2. Caffeine, theophylline and saccharin may bind B2 in the gut and prevent its absorption.

Food sources. Milk, cheese, yogurt, eggs, liver, kidney, fish and beef are all good sources of riboflavin. Other food sources include beans, spinach, avacados, currants, asparagus, broccoli, Brussels sprouts and nuts. Whole-grains or fortified breads are also good sources.

Vitamin B2 is easily destroyed by light. Milk stored in clear glass bottles can lose up to 75 percent of riboflavin in just a few hours. It is important to keep milk away from light as much as possible. Alkaline substances such as sodium bicarbonate, which is used to preserve the bright color of fruits and vegetables, destroy riboflavin. Cooking also causes a partial loss of this vitamin. *Supplemental advice.* Riboflavin should be taken with meals. Because it is water-soluble and easily excreted in the urine, it should be taken in divided doses. Taking large doses all at once does little good. Exercise and dieting may increase the need for riboflavin. Stress, pregnancy and lactation also increase the requirements.

Side effects. Very little vitamin B2 is needed to prevent a deficiency. No side effects or toxicities have been reported with its use. Some interactions with drugs have occurred. Psyllium, alcohol, oral contraceptives and some antibiotics slow the absorption of vitamin B2 in the gut. Caffeine, theophylline and saccharin may bind B2 in the gut and prevent its absorption.

Symptoms of deficiency. A vitamin B2 deficiency is more commonly seen in the elderly and in alcoholics. Signs include an increased sensitivity to light, tearing, tired, burning or itching eyes and fuzzy vision. Symptoms around the mouth include cracks in the corners of the mouth, sore or burning lips, mouth and tongue, and a red/purple swollen tongue. It may hurt to eat or drink, resulting in weight loss. The skin can be affected and there may be flaking or peeling skin around the nose, eyebrows, chin, cheeks, earlobes or hairline. There may also be a rash in the genital area. Some behaioral changes may be seen and include moodiness, nervousness, irritability and depression.

Symptoms of toxicity. There are no known toxicities to vitamin B2. It is a water-soluble vitamin that easily excreted in the urine. It turns the urine a bright yellow color but this is no cause for concern.

Vitamin B3 (Niacin)

Although niacin is needed to maintain a healthy skin, gastrointestinal tract and nervous system, its primary use—in the form of nicotinic acid or inositol hexaniacinate—has been to lower serum lipids and cholesterol. The advantage of niacin in treating high serum cholesterol is that while it lowers other serum lipids, including LDL, it raises the levels of high density lipoprotein (HDL). In this form, it is also used to improve circulation, especially in Raynaud's syndrome or intermittent claudication.

In the form of niacinamide, also called nicotinamide, vitamin B3 has been used to slow the progression of type I diabetes. High doses may even reverse the development of the disease. It may also increases the pancreas' production of insulin. It, along with the other B vitamins is involved in energy metabolism. Because of its effects on the nervous system, vitamin B3 has been used for anxiety, nervousness, depression, insomnia and memory loss. It has also been used for migraine headaches and feeling tired, weak, irritable or depressed. Vitamin B3, in the form of niacinamide, has been used in alcohol dependence, drug-induced hallucinations and schizophrenia.

High-dose niacinamide has been used to relieve the symptoms of rheumatoid arthritis and osteoarthritis. Niacinamide has also been used for diarrhea and improving digestion. It has also been used to improve orgasm.

Food sources. Foods rich in niacin include Torula yeast, brewer's yeast, rice bran, wheat bran and nuts. It is also found in foods high in protein, like chicken, beef and fish. Foods rich in tryptophan, the niacin precursor, include milk, soy, peanuts, eggs, pork, lamb and beef. Niacin is lost in cooking water, but preserved when foods are steamed, baked or stir fried.

Supplemental advice. Vitamin B3 is available in several forms including niacin, nicotinic acid, nicotinate and niacinamide. The therapeutic dose of vitamin B3 ranges from 50 to 3,200 mg per day. A dose of 60 mg of tryptophan is considered to be equal to 1 mg of niacin. Vitamin B3 should be taken with meals to decrease stomach upset.

As much as 1,000 mg have been given to children. For elevated cholesterol, inositol hexaniacinate is the preferred form. Typically, under a doctor's direction of course, 500 mg three times a day is taken for at least two weeks. The dose can then be increased to 1,000 mg three times a day. To treat arthritis, 1,000 mg of niacinamide can be taken three times a day.

Side effects. Vitamin B3 is considered very safe with the major side effect being the uncomfortable flushing of the skin that often occurs at doses greater than 50 mg. Other side effects include headache, nausea, vomiting, dizziness, decreased blood pressure and diarrhea.

Time-released niacin eliminates many of these problems but can cause elevated liver enzymes. Using inositol hexaniacinate generally prevents this as well as flushing. Niacin interacts with the anti-tuberculosis drug, Isoniazid. High doses of inositol hexaniacinate can thin the blood.

Niacin can interfere with the control of blood sugar in those with diabetes and drugs for diabetes may need to be adjusted. It should not be used in people with liver disease. A deficiency of both niacin and tryptophan is characterized by dermatitis, dementia and diarrhea. The skin becomes scaly and dark in places that are exposed to the sun, heat or recurrent trauma. People may have headaches or feel tired, weak, irritable, depressed and have a loss of memory. In a more severe deficiency, symptoms can include disorientation, hysteria and convulsions. Diarrhea, loss of appetite, nausea, indigestion, a red, swollen tongue and ulcers in the mouth may also occur.

Symptoms of deficiency. Niacin deficiencies are most often seen in alcoholics and others with poor diets. Deficiencies can also result from an overactive thyroid gland, pregnancy or liver disease.

Pellagra, a severe deficiency of both niacin and tryptophan, is characterized by dermatitis, dementia and diarrhea. The skin becomes scaly and dark in places that are exposed to the sun, heat or recurrent trauma. The rest of the skin may be very pale. The nervous system is affected as well. People may have headaches or feel tired, weak, irritable, depressed and have a loss of memory. In a more severe deficiency, symptoms can include disorientation, hysteria and convulsions.

The gastrointestinal tract is also affected. Diarrhea results because the cells of lining of the GI tract are not being properly replaced. This may also result in loss of appetite, nausea, indigestion, a red, swollen tongue and ulcers in the mouth. Niacin deficiencies are most often seen in alcoholics and others with poor diets. Deficiencies can also result from an overactive thyroid gland, pregnancy or liver disease. If a deficiency is found, a riboflavin or iron deficiency may be present as well.

Symptoms of toxicity. There are no toxicities to vitamin B3 except the increase in liver enzymes that occurs with high doses. This is reversible if the dose is decreased.

There can be an uncomfortable flushing of the skin that often occurs at doses greater than 50 mg (see above).

Vitamin B5 (pantothenic acid and pantethine; no RDA/DRI established)

Pantothenic acid, a very safe vitamin, is found in just about every food you eat, so it's impossible to be deficient in it. The primary uses of pantothenic acid—also known as calcium pantothenate—is the secretion of hormones, such as cortisone because of the role it plays in supporting the adrenal gland. These hormones assist the metabolism, help to fight allergies and are beneficial in the maintenance of healthy skin, muscles and nerves.

Pantothenic acid is used in the release of energy as well as the metabolism of fat, protein and carbohydrates. It is used in the creation of lipids, neurotransmitters, steroid hormones and hemoglobin. B5 can also lessen the symptoms of rheumatoid arthritis including pain, inflammation and stiffness. It is considered an "anti-stress" vitamin.

It may also be useful for sports related injuries. When used with other B vitamins, vitamin B5 may improve exercise tolerance and delay the onset of fatigue and can aid in wound healing.

Vitamin B5 has been used to treat allergies. It has also been used for ulcerative colitis, aid in the production of red blood cells and support the immune system during infections. Some people believe pantothenic acid is also helpful to fight wrinkles as well as graying of the hair.

Pantethene—the stable form of pantetheine (an active form of pantothenic acid but not pantothenic acid itself)—is used to lower serum cholesterol and triglycerides. Pantothenic acid itself does not have this effect.

Pantothenic acid is found in foods as coenzyme A. It is converted to pantothenic acid during digestion, absorbed, taken up by the cells and made back into coenzyme A. Coenzyme A is needed for the metabolism of fats, proteins and carbohydrates. It is also involved in the synthesis of steroid hormones, the neurotransmitter acetylcholine and vitamin D.

Food sources. The highest concentrations of pantothenic acid are found in brewer's yeast, torula yeast, calf liver, peanuts, mushrooms, soybeans, peas, nuts, broccoli, oranges and sunflower seeds. It is also found in eggs, potatoes, salt water fish, pork and milk. Significant amounts are lost by processing food, including cooking, freezing and canning.

Supplemental advice. Pantothenic acid is usually supplemented as calcium pantothenate. Ten milligrams of calcium pantothenate is equivalent to 9.2 mg of pantothenic acid. Higher amounts are used therapeutically. Pantothenic acid, 250 mg twice daily, will support the adrenal glands and treat allergies. Two grams daily is needed to treat rheumatoid arthritis. Pantethine is used to lower serum cholesterol and triglycerides. The dose is 300 mg three times a day.

Panthethine is expensive compared to niacin or inositol hexaniacinate, other natural cholesterol lowering agents. For this reason, it should be reserved for use in those with diabetes since it does not affect the control of blood sugars as niacin does.

Side effects. There are no side effects, toxicities or interactions with drugs, foods or other supplements.

Symptoms of deficiency. Pantothenic acid is so abundant in nature that a natural deficiency has not been identified. If a pantothenic acid deficiency is artificially created, the major symptom is "burning foot syndrome." Symptoms include numbness and shooting pains in the feet. Fatigue, headache, inflammation and insomnia may be early signs of deficiency. There is also an increased susceptibility to infection.

Symptoms of toxicity. Vitamin B5 is very safe and no toxicity has been identified. Extremely large doses of pantothenic acid have caused diarrhea.

Vitamin B6 (pyridoxine)

Vitamin B6 (also known as pyridoxine, pyridoxine hydrochloride, pyridoxal, pyridoxamine, pyridoxamine-5-phsophate, pyridoxal-5-phosphate, and P-5-P), is considered by many to be the most essential vitamin. It is probably involved in more processes in the body than any other micronutrient. Pyridoxine is required for the balancing of hormonal changes in women as well as assisting the immune system and the growth of new cells. It is also used in the processing and metabolism of proteins, fats and carbohydrates, while assisting with controlling your mood as well as your behavior. Pyridoxine might also be of benefit for children with learning difficulties, as well as assisting in the prevention of dandruff, eczema and psoriasis.

Pyridoxine is used to prevent cardiovascular disease, including atherosclerosis and stroke. Vitamin B6 has been used for symptoms of the nervous system including irritability, autism, convulsions, insomnia and post-partum depression. It is needed to make neurotransmitters in the brain, including serotonin. It is also useful in maintaining healthy nerves in diabetes.

Vitamin B6 reduces the symptoms of multiple sclerosis and in combination with riboflavin (vitamin B2) is used to treat carpal tunnel syndrome. Apgar scores in newborns have been improved with vitamin B6. (See sidebar on next page.)

Pyridoxine is used to reduce the frequency and intensity of asthma attacks. It is needed to make red blood cells and antibodies and has been used for sickle cell disease and to boost immunity. It is also used for recurring kidney stones, diabetes, morning sickness, eczema, premenstrual syndrome, osteoporosis and adverse reactions to MSG.

Pyridoxine is involved in about one hundred enzyme reactions in the body. It works with folic acid and vitamin B12 to help the body process homocysteine, a metabolite of the amino acid methionine. Homocysteine has been linked to an increased risk of atherosclerosis.

In people with vitamin B6 deficiencies who have recurrent kidney stones, pyridoxine, in combination with magnesium, reduces the formation and urinary excretion of calcium oxalate kidney stones. Giving vitamin B6 to people with depression (especially women on oral contraceptives) or women with premenstrual syndrome (PMS) may increase serotonin levels and improve symptoms. B6 may also help clear excess estrogen from the body, again helping to relieve symptoms of PMS.

Pyridoxine is needed to turn iron into hemoglobin and make red blood cells. It is also needed for the body to make antibodies that prevent infections.

Vitamin B6 is needed for the proper growth and for maintenance of most body functions. Rapidly dividing cells, especially those of the immune system, mucous membranes and skin, need pyridoxine. It helps to regulate the activity of steroid hormones and prostaglandins. It is also involved in the regulation of blood sugar through its effect on gluconeogenesis.

Riboflavin and magnesium are needed to convert pyridoxine to pyridoxal-5-phosphate, the active form of vitamin B6 in the body. Vitamin B6 can increase the intracellular levels of magnesium and zinc. Magnesium and riboflavin help increase the absorption of B6.

What Exactly Is the Apgar Score?

Developed in 1952 by Dr. Virginia Apgar's this test measures the infant's physical condition minutes after birth. A score is given for each sign at one minute and five minutes after the birth. If there are problems with the baby an additional score is given at 10 minutes. A score of 7-10 is considered normal, while 4-7 might require some resuscitative measures, and a baby with Apgars of 3 and below requires immediate resuscitation. Playing off Dr. Apgar's name, the letters stand for:

Appearance (Skin Color)
Pulse
Grimace (Reflex Irritability)
Activity (Muscle Tone)
Respiration

Drugs that decrease the levels of pyridoxine or antagonize its effects include oral contraceptives, isoniazid, penicillamine, theophylline and cycloserine. Tobacco, alcohol, air pollutants, hydrazine dyes (FD&C yellow No. 5)) and exposure to radiation have similar effects. A higher intake of vitamin B6 can counteract the antipyridoxine effects of these substances.

Pyridoxine can decrease blood levels of anticonvulsants such as phenytoin and phenobarbital and increase the risk of a seizure.

Food sources. Pyridoxine is found almost exclusively in plant foods, including bananas, walnuts, navy beans, sunflower seeds and wheat germ. Other sources include include spinach, carrots, peas, meat, eggs, chicken, fish and brewer's yeast. Pyridoxal-5-phosphate is found in beef, salmon and chicken. It is affected by heat, oxygen and light and up to 70 percent of vitamin B6 is lost by cooking, processing and refining the food.

Supplemental advice. It is hard to get the RDA/DRI from food so supplements are often necessary. Doses in the range of 30 to 500 mg daily are common. Amounts greater than 50 mg per day should be taken in divided doses throughout the day.

Homocysteine levels can be decreased with 3 mg a day, but 50 mg a day is often recommended. Other therapeutic doses include carpal tunnel syndrome, 50 mg three times a day; PMS, 50 mg twice daily; asthma, 50 mg twice daily; and morning sickness, 30 mg daily.

Symptoms of deficiency. A vitamin B6 deficiency is rare and symptoms are similar to those seen with other B vitamin deficiencies. A severe deficiency is recognized by cracks around the corners of the mouth, ulcers inside the mouth, and a cracked or inflamed tongue. Skin problems resulting from deficiency include eczema, acne and dry scaly skin around the nose, eyes, eyebrows and skin behind the ears. Nervous system problems may include fatigue, insomnia, irritability, confusion and depression. There may be the feeling of pins and needles in the hands and feet. Children may even have seizures. Weight loss, glucose intolerance and frequent colds or other infections may also be noted with low levels of vitamin B6.

Symptoms of toxicity. Vitamin B6 is one of the few water-soluble vitamins associated with some toxicity. Vitamin B6 toxicity occurs when the supplemental pyridoxine overwhelms the liver's ability to add a phosphate group and form the active form of B6, pyridoxal-5-phosphate. Doses up to 100 mg per day are safe for long-term use, but the liver seems to only be able to handle about 50 mg at the time, so dividing the dose is important.

Nerve damage with symptoms of tingling in the feet and loss of muscle coordination are the major symptoms. Toxicity is usually seen when taking greater than 500 mg a day for several months or with short-term use of 2,000 mg a day. Amounts greater than 150 mg per day can suppress lactation. Fortunately, the nerve damage reverses when the vitamin supplement is stopped.

Vitamin B7 (Biotin)

Biotin—sometimes called vitamin H—is necessary for both metabolism and growth in humans. It plays a crucial role in cell growth, the production of fatty acids, metabolism of fats, carbohydrates and proteins into fuel and in niacin (vitamin B3) metabolism. It plays a role in the Krebs cycle, which is the process in which energy is released from food. Biotin is also helpful in maintaining a steady blood sugar level.

Some say biotin can cure baldness—since one of the most visible symptoms of shortage of this vitamin is thinning of hair—and alleviate muscle pain and depression, and function as a cure for dermatitis, although there is no substantial scientific evidence for any of these claims. Biotin is also needed for healthy skin, healthy sweat glands, nerve tissue and bone marrow, and assisting with muscle pain.

It seems that biotin may affect hair color, together with PABA, folic acid and pantothenic acid. Some research had varying results with biotin supplements in returning hair to it original color. This has proved only successful to a limited degree and only when natural vitamins were used, as the synthetic vitamins did not influence the results very much.

The bacteria that normally colonize the colon (large intestine) are capable of making their own biotin. It is not yet known whether humans can absorb a meaningful amount of the biotin synthesized by their own intestinal bacteria.

Food sources. Biotin is present in cheese, beef liver, cauliflower, egg yolk, liver, kidney, mushrooms, chicken breasts, salmon, spinach, brewer's yeast and nuts. It is also manufactured in the body should a small shortage occur.

Supplemental advice. A varied diet should provide enough biotin for most people. Presently, there is no indication that older adults have an increased requirement for biotin. If dietary biotin intake is not sufficient, a daily multivitamin/multimineral supplement will ensure an intake of at least 30 mcg of biotin/day.

Side effects. Individuals on long-term anticonvulsant (anti-seizure) therapy have been found to have reduced levels of biotin in their blood. The anticonvulsants primidone and carbamazepine inhibit biotin absorption in the small intestine. Phenobarbital, phentyoin and carbamazepine appear to increase urinary excretion of biotin. Also, long-term treatment with sulfa drugs or other antibiotics may decrease bacterial synthesis of biotin, potentially increasing the requirement for dietary biotin.

Symptoms of deficiency. Although a shortage of biotin is very rare, it can happen and may result in dry scaly skin, fatigue, loss of appetite, nausea and vomiting, muscle pains, hair loss, anemia, mental depression, tongue inflammation and high cholesterol.

Symptoms of toxicity. No known toxic levels, as excesses are easily lost in the urine and feces. Bodybuilders and athletes consuming raw eggs should be careful of not running into a biotin shortage, since raw eggs contain avidin, which binds with biotin, making it impossible to be absorbed by the body.

Vitamin B9 (folic acid/folate)

The main job for folic acid—the synthetic form of folate—is helping our cells grow and divide properly. It's also important for preventing birth defects. We also need it for making the natural chemicals that control our mood, appetite, and how well we sleep. Folic acid is vital for keeping our arteries open and lowering our chances of a heart attack or stroke.

In 1998, the Institute of Medicine looked at evidence from many new studies and raised the new DRI for folic acid up to 400 mcg for all adults and 600 mcg for pregnant women. The DRIs for children were also raised. Many doctors and nutritionists believe that the adult DRI is still way, way too low. They believe every adult should get at least 400 mcg of folic acid every day, but 800 mcg would be even better.

Even after the RDA for folic acid was lowered, studies show that the average American diet contains only about 200 mcg a day. Not surprisingly, a shortage of folic acid by the new higher DRI is one of the most common vitamin deficiencies, especially among women. One recent study estimated that an astonishing 88 percent of all Americans get less than 400 mcg a day.

In 1992, the U.S. Public Health Service recommended that all women of childbearing age consume 400 mcg of folic acid daily. Every agency and organization concerned with birth defects, from the FDA to the March of Dimes, has strongly endorsed this recommendation. A neural tube defect (NTD) happens when the growing brain, spinal cord and vertebrae (the bones of the spine) of an unborn baby don't develop properly during the first month of pregnancy. The most common NTD is the crippling spina bifida, or "open spine."

Recently, folic acid has been getting a lot of attention for its role in preventing cancer. If you're a woman and get a lot of folic acid in your diet, your chances of colon cancer are sharply lower-by as much as 60 percent. (For some reason, this doesn't work as well for men.) Folic acid may also help prevent cancer of the cervix.

Keeping our artery-damaging homocysteine level low is one of the jobs of folic acid. Working with pyridoxine and cobalamin, folic acid quickly breaks down the homocysteine and removes it from your body before it can do any damage.

Food sources. Folic acid isn't found in that many animal foods, and there's hardly any in milk and other dairy foods. The only good animal sources are chicken liver and beef liver. Beans of all kinds are good sources of folic acid, as is wheat germ. Other good plant sources are spinach and asparagus. Citrus juices and fruits, bananas, cantaloupe, nuts, seeds, liver, dark green leafy vegetables and fortified grain products, such as bread, pasta, breakfast cereals and rice. Half a cup (4 ounces) of cooked spinach contains 130 mcg of folate.

Because most of us don't eat enough beans and fresh vegetables, the FDA has developed rules for fortifying enriched breads, flours, corn meal, rice, noodles, pasta and other grain products with folic acid. As of 1998 all these foods have extra folic acid added to them. The goal is to make sure that everyone gets at least 400 mcg a day from their food.

Supplemental advice. By some estimates, just 1 mg a day could be enough to prevent fifty thousand heart attacks a year. See your doctor before taking folic acid if you have anemia.

Symptoms of deficiency. Individuals in the early stages of folate deficiency may not show obvious symptoms, but blood levels of homocysteine may increase. Lack of folate can also cause anemia.

Symptoms of toxicity. People who take folic acid may develop bright-yellow urine, fever, shortness of breath, a skin rash or, very rarely, diarrhea. Doses over 1,500 mcg/day can cause nausea, appetite loss, flatulence and abdominal distention.

Vitamin B12 (cobalamin)

The most important role of B12 is making healthy red blood cells. When you don't have enough red blood cells to carry oxygen and nutrients around your body, you develop anemia.

Vitamin B12 is synthesized by bacteria in the gut and exists in all foods from animal sources. The stomach secretes a substance called intrinsic factor that is necessary for vitamin B12 to be absorbed. Calcium is also needed for proper absorption to occur.

Vitamin B12 is used with folic acid to prevent heart disease. It is used for nerve pain, ringing in the ear and numbness and tingling in the feet and hands. It helps decrease symptoms of confusion, mood changes, depression and multiple sclerosis in some people. Vitamin B12 is necessary for the body to make red blood cells and keep the immune system functioning.

Vitamin B12 has been used in those with asthma, fatigue, hepatitis, insomnia, epilepsy and infertility. Vitamin B12 is stored in the liver but excess amounts are easily excreted in the urine.

Cobalamin is important in the production of some neurotransmitters, including serotonin and dopamine. Low levels of serotonin have been associated with depression. Low levels of vitamin B12 may result in poor sleep. Vitamin B12 is needed for the secretion of melatonin, a hormone needed for a proper sleep cycle.

Vitamin B12 combines with sulfite and can prevent allergic reactions and asthma in sulfite sensitive people. It is involved in the production of DNA and RNA for cell replication. It is necessary for red blood cell production and for proper immune function.

Methionine is needed for the synthesis of choline. A lack of choline may lead to impaired fatty acid synthesis and a decreased production of myelin, the sheath that covers the nerves, resulting in a nervous system dysfunction.

Nitrous oxide, seizure drugs and alcohol will decrease the levels of vitamin B12 in the blood. People with gastrointestinal diseases that cause absorption problems, including Crohn's disease, ulcers and sprue, may have a vitamin B12 deficiency.

Food sources. Animal sources, including liver and kidney, eggs, fish, cheese and meat are the best sources of vitamin B12. Milk and dairy products are also sources but contain lesser amounts. Plants do not contain the active forms of vitamin B12 unless they are contaminated by bacteria. Vegetarians often eat fermented foods like tempeh and sea vegetables to get vitamin B12 but the body cannot use the form found in these plants.

Vitamin B12 is not stable in the presence of heat, acid or light so care must be taken when cooking and storaging foods.

Supplemental advice. Supplements of vitamin B12 will cover up a folic acid deficiency, so it is important to distinguish between the two before treatment. Vitamin B12 is given with folic acid and B6 to prevent heart disease due to high levels of homocysteine. It might also help prevent anemia, and help treat asthma, fatigue, hepatitis, insomnia, epilepsy and infertility. It is used for problems in the nervous system including nerve pain, ringing in the ear, and numbness and tingling. It is also used in depression, psychosis, irritability, confusion, and mood changes. Vitamin B12 has been used for treating Alzheimer's disease and multiple sclerosis. Since it is important for proper functioning of the immune system, it has been used to slow the progression of HIV to AIDS. Cyanocobalamin is most common oral form of vitamin B12 but must be converted to the active form once absorbed. Hydroxycobalamin is the injectable form.

The injectable form of vitamin B12 is the most common in the United States. The oral tablet is just as effective when given in adequate amounts and malabsorption problems are not present.

Side effects. Vitamin B12 is very safe and is readily excreted in the urine. There are few interactions with vitamin B12. Nitrous oxide, a general anesthetic used primarily during dental procedures, lowers the blood levels. Antiepileptic or seizure drugs and alcohol will also decrease the levels in the blood. People with gastrointestinal diseases that cause absorption problems, including Crohn's disease, ulcers and sprue, may have a vitamin B12 deficiency.

Symptoms of deficiency. Deficiencies are most common in the elderly and alcoholics. Vitamin B12 is stored in the liver, kidney and other body tissues, so a deficiency is rare and is a result of many years of low B12 intake. Symptoms of a B12 deficiency include numbness, pins-and-needles sensations, or a burning feeling in the feet and hands. Fatigue, muscle weakness, confusion, loss of memory and depression are other symptoms. The tongue may be red and inflamed and diarrhea may occur. Heart disease, including high serum cholesterol may be present. Anemia results from low vitamin B12 levels (megaloblastic) or from a lack of intrinsic factor (pernicious) which is needed for B12 absorption from the gut. Deficiencies are most common in the elderly and alcoholics.

Inositol

Inositol plays an important part in the health of cell membranes especially the specialized cells in the brain, bone marrow, eyes and intestines. The function of the cell membranes is to regulate the contents of the cells, which makes effective functioning possible. It may also be of benefit in reducing blood cholesterol levels.

Inositol is said to promote healthy hair and hair growth, to help control estrogen levels and to prevent breast lumps. Men taking extra inositol reported that their hair loss improved, with less hair falling out—although this has not been tested under clinical situations.

Food sources. Inositol is available from both plant and animal sources. Inositol is available from the phytic acid in plants, which can bind with minerals and so affect their absorption negatively. Inositol is available from wheat germ, brewer's yeast, bananas, liver, brown rice, oat flakes, nuts, unrefined molasses, raisins and vegetables.

Supplemental advice. Inositol should be taken in the same amount as the rest of entire B group vitamins. Vitamin E, vitamin C, folic acid and linoleic acid are thought to increase the functioning of inositol.

Side effects. Taking of long-term antibiotics may increase your need for inositol, as well as if you consume a lot of coffee.

Symptoms of deficiency. If your intake of inositol is not sufficient, you may experience symptoms such as eczema, hair loss, constipation and abnormalities of the eyes and raised cholesterol.

Symptoms of toxicity. No toxic effects known, but diarrhea has been noted with the intake of very high dosage of inositol

PABA (para-aminobenzoic acid)

PABA is the shortened name for para-aminobenzoic acid that is often thought of as only an ingredient used in sunscreens to help protect the skin against ultraviolet radiation. However, it is in fact a nutritional ingredient as well.

Since PABA is made in your body from folic acid some health professionals do not consider it a vitamin, but only a B-complex factor.

PABA improves protein use in the body, and it relates to red blood cell formation, as well as assisting the manufacture of folic acid in the intestines. PABA also assists with breaking down of protein, the formation of red blood cells and maintaining intestinal flora.

PABA has been linked to hair growth, as well as reversing the graying of hair, but these results are disappointing. People suffering from vitiligo, over-pigmentation of skin, or without pigment in some spots, have reported an improvement of the skin after more PABA was ingested.

Food sources. PABA is found in liver, kidney, brewer's yeast, molasses, whole grains, mushrooms and spinach. It can also be made by intestinal bacteria.

Supplemental advice. Long-term antibiotic use may require more PABA from the body, but take note of PABA affecting the ability of sulfa drugs. Although not documented in medical terms, some women having problems becoming pregnant claim conceiving after increasing PABA in their diet.

PABA is best used with citamin C and the B vitamins. PABA may make sulfa drugs ineffectual.

Side effects. When higher than factor (SPF) 8 sunscreens are used, the manufacture of vitamin D in the body may be reduced.

Symptoms of deficiency. When PABA is in short supply, fatigue, irritability, nervousness and depression might manifest itself, as well as constipation. Weeping eczema has also been noted in people with PABA deficiency, as well as patchy areas on the skin.

Symptoms of toxicity. Nausea, skin rashes and vomiting might be indicative of PABA taken in excess. Excessive levels of PABA are stored in the body and may cause liver damage.

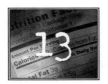

Our Real Needs for Minerals

Like **vitamins, minerals** are also components of enzymes and coenzymes. In addition, minerals are needed to maintain the proper composition of body fluids, to help build bone and make blood cells and to maintain proper nerve function.

There are a variety of important minerals needed to help our bodies function. They are divided into major minerals—needed in larger quantities to maintain health—and trace minerals, which are needed in smaller amounts.

Minerals are stored primarily in the bones and in the muscle tissue. Too much of any one mineral can cause signs of toxicity and may also create an imbalance of others.

The major minerals (those needed in larger amounts) include the following:

- calcium
- phosphorus
- magnesium
- sodium (not on RDA List)
- potassium
- chloride

Calcium, phosphorus and magnesium are important in the development and health of your bones and teeth. Sodium, potassium and chloride—known as electrolytes—are important in regulating the water and chemical balance in our bodies. In addition, your body needs smaller amounts of the following minerals:

• chromium
• copper
• fluouride (not on RDA List)
• iodine
• iron
• manganese
• molybdenum
• selenium (covered in antioxidant chapter)
• zinc (covered in antioxidant chapter)

On the opposite page is chart repeated from Chapter 2. Don't feel you have to study it, though; it can be very confusing, and frankly, not worth all that much.

Here's what you should know about the remaining minerals.

Calcium

Calcium is needed for the formation and maintenance of bones. People often think of bones as a static piece of the body, where very little change occurs, but that is a totally incorrect perception. Bone is a dynamic part of the body and calcium is constantly flowing into, and out of it.

The fact is bone is constantly being regenerated. Children need a lot of calcium because a bone's densest part, the core, is formed during adolescence. Even though the core gets thinner as we age, calcium from foods we eat is deposited on the surface of bones, like rings on a tree. As the rings grow, the bone's diameter expands, and it gets stronger.

Calcium is also necessary for the development of teeth and healthy gums. It is necessary for blood clotting, stabilizes many body functions and is thought to assist in preventing bowel cancer.

It has a natural calming and tranquilizing effect and is necessary for maintaining a regular heartbeat and the transmission of nerve

Table 2.5 Comparisons of RDIs, DRIs, and ULs for Minerals

VITAMIN	Current RDI*	New DRI†	UL‡
Calcium	1000 mg	1300 mg	2500 mg
Iron	18 mg	18 mg	45 mg
Phosphorus	1000 mg	1250 mg	4000 mg
Iodine	150 mcg	150 mcg	1100 mcg
Magnesium	400 mg	420 mg	350 mg§
Zinc	15 mg	11 mg	40 mg
Selenium	70 mg	55 mg	400 mg
Copper	2 mg	0.9 mg	10 mg
Manganese	2 mg	2.3 mg	11 mg
Chromium	120 mcg	35 mcg	ND
Molybdenum	75 mcg	45 mcg	2000 mcg

* The Reference Daily Intake (RDI) is the value established by the Food and Drug Administration (FDA) for use in nutrition labeling. It was based initially on the highest 1968 Recommended Dietary Allowance (RDA) for each nutrient, to assure that needs were met for all age groups.

† The Dietary Reference Intakes (DRI) are the most recent set of dietary recommendations established.

‡ The Upper Limit (UL) is the upper level of intake considered to be safe for use by adults, incorporating a safety factor. In some cases, lower ULs have been established for children.

§ Upper Limit for magnesium applies only to intakes from dietary supplements or pharmaceutical products, not including intakes from food and water.

ND Upper Limit not determined. No adverse effects observed from high intakes of the nutrient.

impulses. It helps with lowering cholesterol, muscular growth, the prevention of muscle cramps and normal blood clotting.

It also helps with protein structuring in DNA and RNA. It provides energy, breaks down fats, maintains proper cell membrane permeability, aids in neuromuscular activity and helps to keep the skin healthy. Calcium also stops lead from being absorbed into bone. Estrogen promotes deposits of calcium in the bones.

Food sources. Milk, milk products, beans, nuts, molasses and fruit contain good amounts of calcium. Fish and seafood, as well as green leafy vegetables including collard greens, kale, and broccoli supply good amounts of calcium. Calcium-enriched fruit juices can also be a good source of this important mineral.

The growing popularity of calcium-fortified foods makes it easier than ever to meet our daily quota without dairy. The 300 mg of calcium in one cup of milk can also be obtained by drinking the same amount of calcium-fortified orange juice or by eating a cup of dried figs or a bowl of certain cereals topped with calcium-enriched soy milk. Just one half-cup of tofu—fortified with calcium sulfate) in a stir-fry—adds a whopping 434 mg of calcium to your day.

Supplemental advice. It is recommended to take one to two parts of calcium and phosphorus to one part of magnesium. Vitamin D and vitamin A are beneficial to have around this nutrient, and it is especially beneficial to take a supplement that is chelated with amino acids.

Side effects. More calcium may be needed if you suffer from osteoporosis, are lacking in Vitamin D, if you have a gum disease or eat processed foods, ingest excess protein, fat, sugar or caffeine, salt or fizzy soda drinks.

Drinking bottled water with a low mineral content could require more dietary calcium and so may the consumption of alcohol, taking a birth control pill, diuretic (water pill) antacids or if you are on hormone replacement therapy.

Phosphorus, sodium, alcohol, coffee and white flour aids the loss of calcium from the body, while too much protein, fat and sugars can have a negative effect with the absorption thereof. Tetracycline and calcium bond together which impairs the absorption of both.

Symptoms of deficiency. Prolonged bone re-absorption from chronic dietary deficiency results in osteoporosis—from either too little bone mass accumulation during growth or higher rate of bone loss at menopause. Dietary calcium deficiency also has been associated with increased risk of hypertension and colon cancer.

When it is in short supply, a variety of symptoms from aching joints, eczema, elevated blood cholesterol, heart palpitations, brittle nails, hypertension (high blood pressure) and insomnia can become evident. Muscle cramps, nervousness, numbness in the arms and legs, rheumatoid arthritis, convulsions, depression and delusions have also been noted.

Symptoms of toxicity. Excess calcium supplementation has been associated with some mineral imbalances such as zinc, but combined with a magnesium deficiency it may cause deposits to form in your kidneys, which could cause kidney stones.

Are You Lactose Intolerant?

Lactose intolerance is the inability to digest significant amounts of lactose, the predominant sugar of milk. This inability results from a shortage of the enzyme lactase, which is normally produced by the cells that line the small intestine. Lactase breaks down milk sugar into simpler forms that can then be absorbed into the bloodstream. When there is not enough lactase to digest the amount of lactose consumed, the results, although not usually dangerous, may be very distressing.

Between thirty and fifty million Americans are lactose intolerant. While not all persons deficient in lactase have symptoms, those who do are considered to be lactose intolerant. Lactose intolerance produces uncomfortable or even painful symptoms after dairy consumption. Common symptoms include nausea, cramps, bloating, gas, and diarrhea, which begin about thirty minutes to two hours after eating or drinking foods containing lactose.

Although milk is currently promoted for one primary nutritional purpose—a source of calcium to slow osteoporosis—calcium can be obtained from other sources. In fact, there is increasing controversy over the merits of calcium obtained from milk for bone density. So do we need to drink milk, or should we shun it?

The Dairy Wars

Clearly, there is consensus that calcium is necessary for good health—but no consensus on whether calcium is best when consumed from dairy or other sources. Supporters say milk is the best source for moving calcium to our bones. Those who disagree, argue that proteins found in dairy products actually rob calcium from bone stores, making plant-based foods, along with exercise, a sounder choice.

One side of the argument claims calcium appears to be drawn from bones to move digested animal protein—regardless of the source—through our bodies. Since the average American's diet is protein-heavy to begin with, they say that eating lots of dairy foods may actually cause people to lose calcium. "When you eat a protein food, such as milk, you may be swallowing calcium, but you turn around and excrete calcium in your urine," said Donna

Herlock, M.D., spokeswoman for the Physicians Committee for Responsible Medicine, a nonprofit advocacy group opposed to milk consumption.

The Harvard Nurses' Health study published in the June 1997 issue of the *American Journal of Public Health* seems to bolster Dr. Herlock's point. The study found that women who ate lots of dairy products had higher rates of bone fractures than women who rarely touched the stuff. It suggested that drinking more milk didn't provide any substantial protection against hip or forearm fractures in middle-aged and older women. "We considered the possibility that dairy protein was responsible for the increase in risk of hip fractures," wrote Diane Feskanich, Sc.D., a professor at Harvard Medical School in Cambridge, Mass., and the study's lead author.

Milk advocates dispute this theory. They say the amount of calcium lost in the urine from drinking a glass of milk is minor compared with the amount of calcium coming in. "For every gram of protein you eat, you lose 1.75 mg of calcium," said Connie Weaver, Ph.D., head of foods and nutrition at Purdue University in Indiana. Using this calculation, since each glass of milk provides 8 grams of protein, you'll lose 14 out of 300 mg of calcium per glass—which doesn't seem like a lot. Since the average American consumes approximately 75 grams of animal protein a day they'd still take in more calcium than they'd lose by drinking just one glass of milk.

Robert Heaney, M.D., a professor of medicine at Creighton University in Omaha, Nebraska, who specializes in bone biology, says milk provides more than just calcium. "The reason why dairy products work is that they contain not only calcium and protein but also phosphorus, magnesium, vitamin D, potassium, and other things associated with good bone health," he said. "It's the logical way to go."

Researchers at the University of Pennsylvania, say exercise during crucial bone-building years is the best predictor of a woman's adult bone health. They tracked the diets and exercise habits of eighty-one girls from age twelve to age eighteen. (Women typically gain 40 percent to 50 percent of their total bone mass during these years.) In the end, those who saw the greatest bone gains were the girls who exercised the most, not those who consumed the most calcium.

"Exercise is more important than calcium," said Thomas Lloyd, Ph.D., lead author of the study. "By age eighteen the game is over. You've got 98 percent of your bone mass," he says. "You may go on to gain 1 percent or 2 percent in your twenties, but it's inconsequential." Both sides make sound arguments for their viewpoints, which only manages to confuse the issue. So, we're back to the original question, should you consume dairy products or not? If it's the calcium you're after, rest assured you can get it from other sources. If you like milk for its flavor—or out of force of habit—go ahead and drink it. But, to minimize dangerous fat, I advise you to drink the skim version. Granted, it's an acquired taste, but once you're used to it—which won't take long—whole milk will seem overly sweet and heavy to you.

Phosphorus

Phosphorus is an essential mineral that is required by every cell in the body for normal function. Approximately 85 percent of the body's phosphorus is found in bone. Phosphorus is present in the body and can be found mainly in the bones and muscles—at a total body content of around 400–500 grams.

Phosphorus is very involved with bone and teeth formation as well as most metabolic actions in the body, including kidney functioning, cell growth and the contraction of the heart muscle.

The main inorganic component of bone is calcium phosphate salts while cell membranes are composed largely of phospholipids. While it assists the body in vitamin use—especially some B group vitamins—it also is involved in converting food to energy.

Some scientists are concerned about the increasing amounts of phosphates in the diet which can be attributed to phosphoric acid in soft drinks and phosphate additives in a number of commercially prepared foods. Because phosphorus is not as tightly regulated by the body as calcium, blood phosphate levels can rise slightly with a high phosphorous diet, especially after meals.

High blood phosphate levels reduce the formation of the active form of vitamin D (calcitriol) in the kidneys, reduce blood calcium, and lead to increased PTH release by theparathyroid glands. However, high blood phosphorus levels also lead to decreased urinary calcium excretion. If sustained, elevated PTH levels could have an adverse effect on bone mineral content, but this effect has only been observed in humans on diets that were high in phosphorus and low in calcium.

Food sources. Phosphorus is found in most foods because it is a critical component of all living organisms. Dairy products, meat, and fish are particularly rich sources of phosphorus. Other sources include eggs, seeds, broccoli, apples, carrots, asparagus, bran, brewer's yeast and corn. Phosphorus is also a component of many polyphosphate food additives, and is present in most carbonated soft drinks as phosphoric acid.

Supplemental advice. Calcium and phosphorus must be taken in balance or a deficiency might be formed. If calcium is in short supply relative to phosphorus there may be increased risks of high blood pressure and bowel cancer.

Vitamins D and A, as well as iron, manganese, protein and unsaturated fatty acids, increase the effectiveness of phosphorus.

When more may be required, aluminum hydroxide used in antacids may interfere with the absorption of phosphorus but a deficiency is most unlikely, as phosphorus is so abundant in our everyday diet.

Symptoms of deficiency. Deficiency of this element is unusual but may have symptoms varying from painful bones, irregular breathing, fatigue, anxiety, numbness, skin sensitivity and changes in body weight. A ratio of 2:1 in the diet between phosphorus and calcium can cause low blood calcium levels.

Symptoms of toxicity. Ingesting dosages of phosphorus exceeding 3 to 4 grams may be harmful as it can interfere with calcium absorption, such as the high level in fizzy soda drinks.

Magnesium

Magnesium plays an important role in at least three hundred fundamental enzymatic reactions and therefore is of vital importance in our health. Magnesium helps with formation of bone and teeth and assists the absorption of calcium and potassium. Where calcium stimulates the muscles, magnesium is used to relax the muscles. It is further needed for cellular metabolism and the production of energy through its help with enzyme activity. It is used for muscle tone of the heart and assists in controlling blood pressure.

Together with vitamin B 12, it helps prevent calcium oxalate kidney stones. It helps prevent depression, dizziness, muscle twitching, and pre-menstrual syndrome. It can help prevent the calcification of soft tissue and may help prevent cardiovascular disease, osteoporosis, and certain forms of cancer, and it may reduce cholesterol levels.

Magnesium assists the parathyroid gland to process vitamin D, and a shortage here can cause absorption problems with calcium. It is also used for the management of premature labor, and for the prophylaxis and treatment of seizures in toxemia of pregnancy.

Magnesium is being investigated for the treatment of migraine headaches.

Food sources. Magnesium is found in dairy products, fish, meat and seafood, as well as in legumes, apples, apricots, avocados, bananas, whole grain cereals, nuts, dark green vegetables, and cocoa, while hard water and mineral water may also supply it in fair quantities.

Supplemental advice. Magnesium is best taken with calcium, iron, B group vitamins as well as vitamin E. It has been found that people under stress have low magnesium levels, indicating that magnesium may be beneficial to those under stress.

Side effects. Consumption of alcohol, diuretics, high levels of zinc and vitamin D may increase your magnesium requirement. This will also apply if you are taking diuretics (water pills), have diarrhea or perspiring heavily as well as taking large amounts of vitamin C.

Symptoms of deficiency. A severe deficiency caused by malabsorption, chronic alcoholism, renal dysfunction, or the use of certain medications can cause neuromuscular manifestations, and personality changes can occur.

Many cardiovascular problems are indicated with magnesium in short supply and rapid heartbeats as well as fatigue, irritability, and seizure can occur. Insomnia, poor memory, painful periods, depression, hypertension and confusion may also be indicative of magnesium in short supply.

A deficiency may also be a contributing factor to incontinence in older people and bedwetting in children.

Symptoms of toxicity. If you have kidney or heart problems, check with your medical practitioner before taking a magnesium supplement as an over supply can in severe cases lead to coma and death.

Sodium (not on RDA List)

Sodium is an electrolyte in the body and is required in the manufacture of hydrochloric acid in the stomach, which protects the body from any infections that may be present in food. Sodium is required by the body, but most people have a far too high intake of sodium (salt) in their diet. The fact is, we get enough sodium from the foods we eat. Yet, we add to this amount when we eat chips fries, and other prepared foods.

Food sources. Sodium is found in table salt, anchovies, bacon, fast foods, processed foods and snack foods. The best advice is to read labels on packaged and canned goods. Preserved and processed foods make excessive use of salt in the preparation of the foods, and although you might not be adding extra salt to these products, they are already loaded with sodium.

Supplemental advice. People consuming large amounts of sodium, should look at ingesting extra potassium to balance it. Additional magnesium and calcium is also advised. People taking lithium for the control of bipolar depression should not be on a sodium restricted diet—but please discuss this with your medical practitioner. A person should consume about half the amount of sodium in relation to potassium and is best taken with vitamin D.

If you perspire a lot, do not take salt tablets. They are unnecessary and can be dangerous.

Symptoms of deficiency. A deficiency is rare, but can easily happen with diarrhea, vomiting or excessive sweating, and a shortage may lead to nausea, dizziness, poor concentration and muscle weakness.

Symptoms of toxicity. Excessive sodium may cause high blood pressure, which may lead to a host of health problems. Excessive long-term use of sodium may also cause a loss of calcium from your body.

Potassium

Potassium is one of the electrolytes we all require to maintain health. It is needed for growth, building muscles, transmission of nerve impulses and heart activity. Potassium, together with sodium—potassium inside the cell and sodium in the fluid surrounding the cell—work together for the nervous system to transmit messages as well as regulating the contraction of muscles.

Food sources. Potassium is found in fruit, vegetables as well as whole grains, citrus fruit, molasses, fish and unprocessed meats. Potassium is well absorbed but is not stored in large quantities in the body. Potassium is lost from food when canning. If you suffer from kidney stones, you might benefit from increasing high potassium containing foods in your diet to supply more potassium to your body, as higher potassium levels have proved helpful in preventing kidney stones.

Supplemental advice. Potassium is easily lost in the urine, and if large amounts of salt is ingested, it may be wise to take a potassium supplement. If you suffer from diabetes or kidney problems, do not take a potassium supplement without your doctor's consent. A person should take twice as much potassium as sodium. Potassium is best taken with vitamin B6.

If you are into bodybuilding, it is also a good idea to increase your potassium intake, since potassium is needed to maintain your muscles in good form, controlling your muscle actions, and since potassium is lost in excessive sweating and urine. A great way to include this in your diet is to have a banana, citrus fruit or even a dash of apple cider vinegar.

Side effects. If you are suffering from vomiting, diarrhea or extreme sweating, you may require more potassium or if your diet includes mostly processed foods, large amounts of caffeine, alcohol, or if you take diuretic pills or laxatives.

Symptoms of deficiency. The kidneys excrete any excesses, but deficiencies are seldom found in people on normal diets, although most people could look at increasing their potassium intake. A deficiency may result in fatigue, cramping legs, muscle weakness, slow reflexes, acne, dry skin, mood changes, irregular heartbeat.

Symptoms of toxicity. Excessive potassium can be toxic and will affect your heart but is mainly a problem when you suffer from a problem such as kidney failure.

Chloride

Chloride—not to be confused with chlorine—is formed when chlorine gas dissolves in water but is also a dietary mineral needed by the body for optimum health. Chloride in the diet works with potassium and sodium, the two electrolytes, to control the flow of fluid in blood vessels and tissues, as well as regulating acidity in the body, and also forms part of hydrochloric acid in the stomach.

A high concentration of chloride in the body may result in fluid retention, but sodium is normally the culprit for the retention.

Food sources. Table salt and salty foods, such as olives, are the most concentrated sources of chloride. Table salt is known chemically as sodium chloride. Chloride is also found in moderate amounts in meats, chicken, fish, grains, fruits, vegetables, especially tomatoes, nuts, milk products and seeds.

Supplemental advice. There is no need for supplemental chloride. The chlorine in tap water, used for purification, normally evaporates when boiled.

Symptoms of deficiency. A deficiency of chloride is extremely rare and unlikely to occur but a deficiency of chlorine in the body may cause excessive loss of potassium in the urine, weakness and lowered blood pressured. When you suffer from vomiting, diarrhea and excessive sweating you might be in need of extra chlorine.

Food sources. Chloride is found in table salt as well as kelp, olives, tomatoes, celery and other foods.

While the amounts of the following minerals our bodies need are very small, they are still important.

Chromium

Chromium is an essential nutrient required for normal sugar and fat metabolism. It is present in the entire body but with the highest concentrations in the liver, kidneys, spleen and bone. Chromium is necessary for energy production, and it maintains stable blood sugar levels. In cooperation with other substances, it controls insulin as well as certain enzymes. It works with GTF (Glucose Tolerance Factor) when this hormone-affiliated agent enters the bloodstream because of an increase of insulin in the bloodstream.

GTF—containing niacin, vitamin B3, glycine, cysteine, glutamic acid—enhances insulin, which results in the sugars passing quicker into the cells and in that way they are removed from the bloodstream. By stabilizing the blood sugar level it also assists in regulating the cholesterol in the blood.

Natural chromium levels decline with age and so with the action of the GTF. Although chromium picolinate is readily absorbed by the body (and is one of the best types of chromium when it comes to absorption), it will only be absorbed it if there is a shortage of chromium. Chromium picolinate is chromium chelated with picolinate—a natural amino acid metabolite and is helpful in assisting with the loss of fat and increased lean muscle tissue. Chromium picolinate in this form is the most bio-available. Avoid chromium chloride, which is found in some supplements. It is mostly unabsorbable.

Food sources. Chromium is found in eggs, beef, whole grains, brewer's yeast as well as molasses. Chromium absorption is made more difficult when milk, as well as when foods high in phosphorus are eaten at the same time.

Supplemental advice. If you are overweight, have high cholesterol, exercise heavily or have sugar cravings, you might benefit from a chromium supplement. It is best taken with vitamin B3, glycine, cysteine and glutamic acid. Chromium picolinate has been used as a carbohydrate-burning supplement for some time and has proved very successful. It is also required in synthesis of fats, protein, and carbohydrates and may assist in preventing coronary artery disease. If you are diabetic, do not supplement with chromium, as it can make your blood sugar levels drop. Some people have reported a skin rash and lightheadedness—if this occurs, stop taking the supplement and consult your medical practitioner.

Symptoms of deficiency. A shortage of chromium may also lead to anxiety, fatigue, glucose intolerance (particularly in people with diabetes), inadequate metabolism of amino acids, and an increased risk of arteriosclerosis.

Symptoms of toxicity. Because chromium is not easily absorbed (chromium picolinate is the best absorbed) and since it is lost easily in the urine, toxicity does not seem to be a problem, but dermatitis has been noted, as well as gastrointestinal ulcers and liver and kidney damage if taken in large dosages over prolonged periods.

Copper

Copper is required in the formation of hemoglobin, red blood cells as well as bones, while it helps with the formation of elastin as well as collagen—making it necessary for wound healing. A lack of copper can lead to increased blood fat levels. It is also necessary for the manufacture of the neurotransmitter noradrenaline as well as for the pigmentation of your hair.

Copper and zinc absorption are closely related. Although copper is also needed in relatively small amounts, research is being conducted to determine the optimum need of this mineral. It is known that if large amounts of copper are present, then zinc and vitamin C are reduced in the body; and large amounts of vitamin C and zinc can negatively influence the level of copper in the body. Also, large amounts of fructose can make a copper deficiency worse.

Copper can be stored in the body, and daily intake in the diet is not necessary. Copper is best absorbed and utilized in the body when cobalt, iron, zinc and folic acid are available.

Food sources. Copper is made available from a variety of foods, such as whole grain, liver, molasses, and nuts, but water from copper pipes will also carry copper in it, and copper cooking utensils will also add more copper to be ingested.

Supplemental advice. Should extra zinc supplements be taken, your need for copper may be increased.

Side effects. Be careful of having any liquids stored in copper containers, as the liquid could have absorbed too much of the copper.

Symptoms of deficiency. If copper is deficient in the body, iron is also normally in short supply, leading to anemia as well as the likelihood for infections, osteoporosis, thinning of bones, thyroid gland dysfunction, heart disease as well as nervous system problems.

Symptoms of toxicity. Toxic levels will lead to diarrhea, vomiting, liver damage as well as discoloration of the skin and hair, while mild excesses will result in fatigue, irritability, depression and loss of concentration and learning disabilities. Children getting too much copper may have hyperactive tendencies.

Fluoride (not on RDA List)

About half of all U.S. residents drink fluoridated water. Fluorine is a constituent of bones and teeth. It is beneficial in most cases in preventing dental cavities, but the addition of fluoride to drinking water is a controversial subject. (The dosage determined to prevent dental cavities is 1 mg Fl/L.)

While fluoridated water has helped reduce the amount of tooth decay among children in the U.S., more is not necessarily better. People who get too much fluoride from a variety of sources can have permanently discolored teeth.

Food sources. It is found in seafood, tea, tap water as well as the food grown in areas where fluorine is present in the soil and water.

Supplemental advice. Don't take fluoride supplements without consulting a local physician or dentist.

Side effects. There is some evidence that it is effective in the treatment of osteoporosis. Although results are preliminary, researchers found an increase in the retention of calcium was accompanied by a reduction of bone demineralization, after treatment with fluorine salts.

Symptoms of deficiency. Fluoride deficiency weakens the enamel of the teeth, often resulting in increased dental cavities.

Symptoms of toxicity. Excess fluoride stains the teeth with mottled spots—known as dental fluorosis.

Iodine

Iodine is used in the production of hormones (such as thyroxine, thyroxin) by the thyroid gland, which in turn regulates the conversion of fat to energy, stabilizing our body weight as well as controlling our cholesterol levels. These hormones produced from iodine are also needed to help form our bones, as well as keeping our skin, nails, hair and teeth in prime condition. Some indication also exists that iodine is helpful in preventing cancer of the breast and womb. Iodine is also thought to help protect the thyroid from the effects of radiation, and the Polish government handed out iodine tablets to their population after the explosion at Chernobyl.

Food sources. Iodine in our food is dependant on the iodine found in the ground where the food is grown, in the food the animals receive, as it influences the iodine content in the meat and eggs we consume. Iodine is found in eggs, milk, sea fish and sea food, and sea vegetables, such as kelp and asparagus.

If you have an underactive thyroid try and avoid large amounts of raw cabbage, peaches, pears, spinach and Brussels sprouts as they may block the absorption of iodine.

Supplemental advice. When iodine in the soil is very low, or if very little seafood is consumed a person may want to check their iodine intake, or when breast feeding or pregnant as well as being on a sea-salt restricted diet.

Side effects. If your diet is supplemented with too much kelp or iodine you could have problems with acne or skin rashes.

Symptoms of deficiency. Iodine is not stored in the body, but various items in our diet do supply iodine, so a shortage does not happen quickly. When iodine is deficient the thyroid gland enlarges (referred to as a goiter) to maximize the amount of iodine to be extracted from the blood. If this problem is not corrected, a shortage of this hormone in the body may lead to constipation, obesity, weakness, mental slowness as well as mental problems. Goiter is rare in the U.S.

Symptoms of toxicity. Although too low levels of iodine can cause a goiter, so too can an overly high intake of iodine

Iron

Iron is an essential element carrying oxygen, forming part of the oxygen-carrying proteins—hemoglobin in red blood cells and myoglobin in muscles. It is also a component of various enzymes and is concentrated in bone marrow, the liver, and the spleen.

The production of hemoglobin and myoglobin (the form of hemoglobin found in muscle tissue) requires this nutrient. It is also needed for the oxygenation of red blood cells, a healthy immune system and for energy production.

Iron absorption is negatively affected when oxalic acid—found in spinach, Swiss chard, tea, coffee, and soy—are consumed. Antacid medication, coffee and tea drinkers at mealtimes, people on calorie restricted diets and women with a heavy flow during menstruation may require more iron. Try to cut out tea and coffee at mealtimes to minimize their interference with iron absorption.

Food sources. Heme iron (present in red blood cells and muscles) found in meat, poultry and fish—is readily absorbed; Non-heme iron, with the absorption more influenced by other dietary factors, is present in cereals, fruits, grains, beans and vegetables.

Supplemental advice. Iron supplements should not be taken together with calcium, zinc or vitamin E if in the form of ferrous sulfate. Iron should be taken between meals with Vitamin C, while manganese, copper, molybdenum, vitamin A and the B group are also beneficial. Iron in a supplement should be almost balanced with zinc.

Large iron supplementation can contribute to the hardening of arteries, heart disease and reducing zinc absorption.

Side effects. Some research being conducted is to test the possibility of high iron stores in the body being responsible for an increased risk of chronic diseases, such as cancer and heart disease, through oxidative mechanisms.

Symptoms of deficiency. Severe iron deficiency results in anemia and in red blood cells that have a low hemoglobin concentration. Anemia in pregnancy increases the risk of having a premature baby or a baby with low birth weight.

In young children, iron deficiency can manifest in behavioral abnormalities (including reduced attention), reduced cognitive performance and slow growth. In adults, severe iron deficiency anemia impairs physical work capacity.

Other symptoms of deficiency may include fatigue, poor stamina, intestinal bleeding, excessive menstrual bleeding, nervousness, heart palpitations and shortness of breath. It may also cause your mouth corners to crack, brittle hair, difficulty in swallowing, digestive disturbances and spoon shaped nails with ridges running lengthwise.

Symptoms of toxicity. High iron content in the body has been linked to cancer and heart disease. People of European origin, sometimes have a genetic abnormality for storing excessive iron (about one in three hundred people) where ten percent of these populations carry a gene for hemochromatosis.

Iron supplements are the leading cause of death in children—so keep the supplements out of the reach of children. A fatal dose for children could be as little as 600 mg. Iron can be poisonous and if too much is taken over a long period could result in liver and heart damage, diabetes and skin changes.

Manganese

Manganese is one of those oft-overlooked trace elements, even though it is essential to our health. It enables our bodies to utilize vitamin C, B1, biotin as well as choline. It is used in the manufacture of fat, sex hormones and breast milk in females. It is thought to also help neutralize free radicals as well as being of assistance in preventing diabetes and needed for normal nerve function.

Manganese also stimulates growth of the connective tissue and is also thought to be of importance in brain functioning. Manganese is lost in milling and absorption is also negatively influenced in the presence of large amounts of calcium, phosphorous, zinc, cobalt and soy protein. Manganese is depleted in the soil by extensive use of chemical fertilizers or too much lime, and food grown in such soil will have a low manganese content.

Food sources. It is found in nuts, avocados, eggs, brown rice, spices, whole grains, leafy greens as well as tea and coffee.

Supplemental advice. Manganese is best taken with vitamins B1, E, and calcium, as well as phosphorous. A higher intake may be necessary when breast-feeding or when taking a calcium or phosphorous supplement.

Symptoms of deficiency. Deficiencies are rare but would include poor bone growth, problems with the disks between the vertebrae, birth defects and problems with blood glucose levels and reduced fertility. Serious deficiency in children can result in paralysis, deafness and blindness.

Symptoms of toxicity. Toxicity by diet is rare. Miners who are exposed to high levels of manganese, which can also be inhaled, can experience a side effect known as "manganese madness."

Molybdenum

Molybdenum is a component of three different enzymes, which is involved in the metabolism of nucleic acids—DNA and RNA—

iron as well as food into energy. These three enzymes are sulfite oxidase, xanthine oxidase and aldehyde oxidase.

Molybdenum assists in the breaking down of sulfite toxin build-ups in the body and may prevent cavities. With these qualities, there might be evidence of antioxidant properties in this nutrient. It assists the body by fighting the nitrosamines, which are associated with cancer, and may help to prevent anemia. It is needed for normal cell function and nitrogen metabolism.

Food sources. Milk, lima beans, spinach, liver, grain, peas and other dark green leafy vegetables contain molybdenum.

Supplemental advice. If your diet consists mainly of refined foods or if you are taking copper supplements, you might be running low on molybdenum.

An excess of copper, tungsten and sulfates can deplete molybdenum. Heat and moisture change supplemental molybdenum.

Side effects. Molybdenum deficiencies in older males have also been linked to impotence and may be of value in fighting mouth and gum disorders. Molybdenum is part of sulfite oxidase, an enzyme that breaks down sulfites. Sulfites are found in protein food as well as chemical preservatives in certain foods and drugs. Should your body not be able to break down these sulfites, a toxic build-up results, and your body may have an allergic reaction. These reactions can be respiratory problems such as asthma.

Symptoms of deficiency. Deficiencies of molybdenum are identified by the absence of the three molybdenum enzymes. The deficiency of this element and the metabolic disorders are accompanied by abnormal excretion of sulfur metabolites, low uric acid concentrations, and elevated hypoxanthine and xanthine excretion.

The absences of sulfite oxidase in metabolic disorder can lead to death at an early age. High rates of esophageal cancer have been reported in regions where the soil levels of molybdenum are low as well as vitamin C intake—although this does not clinically prove that molybdenum might be involved with prevention of certain cancers.

Symptoms of toxicity. Dosages of more than 15 mg may be toxic and excess molybdenum in the body can interfere with the metabolism of copper in the body, can give symptoms of gout, and may cause diarrhea, anemia and slow growth.

Selenium

Selenium is a powerful antioxidant that works to protect cells from damage, important for cell growth. Selenium is currently being investigated for its potential to prevent cancer. (For a detailed discussion of selenium see Chapter 9.)

Zinc

Zinc is an antioxidant necessary for a healthy immune system and is also of use in fighting skin problems such as acne, boils and sore throats. It is also needed for cell division and is needed by the tissue of the hair, nails and skin to be in top form. Zinc is further used in the growth and maintenance of muscles. (For a detailed discussion of zinc see Chapter 9.)

There are a few other nonessential minerals found in our diets that aren't listed in the RDA/DRI lists. Here is a quick summary:

Boron

Because of its affinity to calcium and magnesium, boron is used to help with menopausal symptoms, as well as maintaining healthy bones. Boron enhances the body's ability to use calcium, magnesium, as well as vitamin D. It also seems to assist in brain functioning and recognition. Boron seems to prevent calcium and magnesium from being lost in the urine and may help with decreasing menstrual pain by increasing the oestradiol level, which is a very active type of estrogen. People have also reported the reduction of arthritis symptoms with an intake of boron.

Boron food sources include prunes, dates, raisins, honey, nuts, fresh fruit such as grapes and pears, green leafy vegetables and beans.

Cobalt

Cobalt is part of the vitamin B12 molecule. It is required in the manufacture of red blood cells and in preventing anemia. An excessively high intake of cobalt may damage the heart muscles and may cause an over-production of red blood cells or damage to the thyroid gland. Cobalt is present in a variety of vegetables.

Silicon

Silicon is used to keep bones, cartilage, tendons and artery walls healthy and may be beneficial in the treatment of allergies, heartburn and gum disease, as well as assisting the immune system. It is also required by the nails, hair and skin to stay in good condition and is useful in counteracting the effects of aluminum.

Silicon is not present in the body in large amounts, yet is found in virtually every type of tissue in the body. Do not confuse it with silicone. Silicon is also called silica and is a natural substance while silicone is a man-made industrial polymer used in breast enlargement operations.

Silicon is present in onions, wheat, oats, millet, barley, rice, beetroot and alfalfa, as well as leafy green vegetables and whole grains. Silicon levels drop as we age, and it might, therefore, be beneficial as an anti-aging component in our diets.

Sulfur

Sulfur, an acid-forming, nonmetallic element, is not treated as an essential mineral since there are no specific deficiency symptoms. Although sulfur might not be an essential mineral, it is an essential element of protein, biotin and vitamin B1. It is part of the chemical structure of the amino acids methionine, cysteine, taurine and glutathione. It is also necessary in the synthesis of collagen, which is needed for good skin integrity.

Sulfur is found in the hair, nails and skin. Sulfur is about as common in the body as better-known nutrients like potassium. Sulfur is used to detoxify the body, to assist the immune system and to fight the effects of aging and age-related illnesses such as arthritis. Sulfur is normally found in protein foods, such as eggs, garlic, lettuce, cabbage and Brussels sprouts.

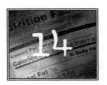

Bottom Line? It's Up to Us

Ronald versus Andy. When I was a boy, my wise mother knew how to get me to eat broccoli. All she had to say was, "But Michael, it's Andy Boy's." Andy was a likeable, animated character akin to Buster Brown who—those old enough to remember—lived in our shoes. Andy Boy, you see, loved broccoli and promoted it unabashedly.

As I grew bigger and stronger—partially due to my broccoli consumption, I'm sure—and approached puberty, I developed a thing for another food character named Chiquita. Thanks to her, my banana intake increased. Both Andy Boy and Chiquita's popularity declined a couple of decades ago, coinciding with the emergence of a clown named Ronald—backed by a seemingly unlimited advertising budget. Ronald promised kids fun while they consumed a tasty diet heavy in fat, salt and sugar.

It seems Ronald's creators learned a few tricks from Andy and Chiquita. Faced with a myriad of eating choices, they recognized strong brand image paved the way for product or brand domination. Spending millions promoting Ronald also helped, of course.

By the way, I've heard Andy Boy and Chiquita Banana are still around. The last I heard they were rumored to be singing karaoke duets in seedy motel lounges near airports. The ageless Ronald, of course, is still going strong.

Then and Now

When you look at photographs snapped in the 1940s, '50s, and '60s, you notice a big difference. Besides the funky clothes and cars, everyone was thin. And, they did it before there were food pyramids, RDAs and DRIs!

There are a number of reasons for this chronic thinness. People were more active then, both at their jobs, at home and during leisure time. But the biggest reason has to do with eating habits. There were no low-cost fast food restaurants—in fact eating out was a special treat, certainly not a daily occurrence.

Back then, food was more of a necessity and took a greater portion of the family budget. People were more apt to eat to live. Today, many of us live to eat, and there's plenty of encouragement for us to do so.

It starts with advice for when we first wake up until we go to sleep. Breakfast cereals and sticky cinnamon rolls, late-night drive-through windows at the burger joint. Though they swear up and down they don't deliberately market to children, food corporations bypass parents and speak directly to impressionable children in order to seduce them—with their parents tagging along—into buying and eating their products. The result is a fattening of America where thirty-five percent of adults, 12 percent of adolescents, and 14 percent of children in the United States are overweight and experience the health risks that entails.

"Nobody can say that these foods in reasonable quantities are bad," said Dr. Marion Nestle. "Hamburgers have nutrients; milkshakes have nutrients, but they are very high in calories. And people don't even notice the 'eat-more' message in the ads." It's a sad state of affairs when the most frequent food consumed to fulfill our daily vegetable requirement is potatoes—usually as chips and French fries.

I hate to break the news, but as much as the food manufactures love you and your money, your health is not their number-one concern. Just as we farm out our lawn mowing, dry cleaning and childcare, we've assigned our nutrition duty to government agencies and food companies. And what have they come up with? Ambiguous, lobby-influenced guidelines based on sample data geared towards average healthy people. The result? Consumer confusion and frustration.

st of items checked out.
ucker Library

ustomer ID: **********9108

tle: Real RDAs for real people : why "off
): 32071025934640
ue: 09/28/16

tle: **Adult Paperback
): 32071000000250
ue: 09/28/16

>tal items: 2
>tal fines: $4.35
'7/2016 3:38 PM
1ecked out: 23
verdue: 0
>ld requests: 0
:ady for pickup: 0

> renew call TeleCirc: 404-508-6900
r visit our website at
ww.dekalblibrary.org

I talked about this before, but I believe it bears repeating. Representatives for every food type, whether representing a food commodity or a brand, have lobbyists to "work with" Congress and any government agency involved with food; in particular, the Food and Drug Administration and the U.S. Department of Agriculture. They help influence and mold legislation favorable to their clients and perform damage control to keep unfavorable news from swaying government policy.

But their influence doesn't stop there. I talked about these issues in depth earlier, but I'll talk about them some more. Besides influencing government, they also . . .

• sponsor research and report only positive results.
• set up or financially support trade associations with official-sounding but evasive names.
• hire scientists and nutritionists to not only boost the nutritional value of their products but keep them from "testifying for the opposition."
• fund cash-strapped researchers and research institutions.
• support official meetings, conferences, medical and nutritional journals and professional societies.
• when necessary, file lawsuits to silence critics (see Oprah Winfrey).

Frankly, it is virtually impossible for nutritional experts and organizations *not* to be involved with the food industry, since they are more than willing to defray costs, and it helps promote their products. Problems arise when industry sponsorship influences research results and opinions. Sometimes it's impossible to tell.

Sometimes, the shoe is slipped on the other foot. Take the well-known and well-respected American Heart Association (AHA). In 1988, the AHA started a program called "Heart-Healthy," in which the AHA allowed food companies to put a special label on food packages that met their criteria for preventing heart disease. Sounds innocent enough, until you learn the AHA was charging a $40,000 fee for testing products and an "education fee" which could run up to $1 million. Under pressure, they later rolled back the fees and modified the program, but not entirely. Today many AHA "approved" products bearing a "Heart-Checked" label include Fruity Marshmallow Krispies and Frosted Flakes.

Although it might seem I've painted an ugly picture of scallywags trying their hardest to sabotage our health, it's not that simple. Everyone involved in the food industry, be they lobbyists, researchers or company executives, believes in what they're doing and saying. While that might be true, you better believe their self-interest will trump ours every time.

The Net Result

While the federal Dietary Guidelines for Americans are supposed to provide nutritional advice to keep Americans healthy, their "one-size-fits-all" approach to diet poorly addresses the health needs of us all, especially the traditional eating habits and genetic makeup of African Americans and other racial minorities. For example, compared to Caucasians, African Americans have much more lactose intolerance, hypertension, diabetes, cancer and obesity.

I'm not pining for the good old days of skinny people. Back then we didn't know the dangers from substances such as lead-based paint, tobacco and asbestos. Face, it as far as health is concerned, we're much better off than decades ago. Due to medical advances and improved diagnosis and treatment, life expectancy has steadily increased. Yet, many of us seem willing to throw it all away and damage our health by overeating and gorging ourselves on highly processed and refined foods.

Maybe it's because were frustrated by the conflicting information and many of us are thoroughly confused. Take dairy products for example. Milk and related products are firmly implanted in our brains as necessary to build strong bones, yet not everyone agrees.

Despite the increasing prevalence of obesity in America, the government's new guidelines did not cut back on recommended servings of meat, cheese and other fatty foods, says Neal D. Barnard, M.D., president of Physicians Committee for Responsible Medicine. "Rather than encourage Americans to eat right, our public officials cater to the meat and dairy lobbies," he says. It's also helpful if you know what axes Dr. Bernard and PCRM are grinding. They are champions of vegetarianism and often fight for animal rights issues.

Maybe Some of Us Are in Denial

Of course what we eat is our business, but companies selling food should spend as much money on unbiased health research as they do on lobbyists and advertising. Frankly, despite what you're told via slick ads, it is not our patriotic duty to drink soda pop.

Not all the blame can be placed on the food industry and those who try to influence it. When 1,450 employed adults were surveyed by Oxford Health Plans as to the state of their health, 17 percent described it as "excellent" and in the same breath admitted to one or more of these dubious habits:

- 55 percent were at least 25 pounds overweight
- 36 percent never exercised
- 31 percent smoked
- 29 percent drank at least four cups of coffee or tea a day
- 26 percent were likely to eat salty or sugary snacks
- 25 percent did not eat a healthy breakfast
- 24 percent were likely to eat fried foods
- 21 percent drank at least three glasses of alcohol a day

"Denial is dangerous when it comes to your health," said Alan Muney, executive vice president of Oxford Health in news release announcing the survey. "It exacts a heavy toll down the road." "So what?" You might ask. Well, the survey also shows health habits do affect our work. For example, people with healthy habits . . .

- feel the most motivated at work
- feel the most useful on the job
- feel the least amount of workplace stress
- are less likely to lose sleep over their jobs
- are least likely to miss personal or family activities due to work

Those who think they are in excellent health but admit to the worst health habits . . .

- are most likely to sit at their desks all day
- don't take breaks at work
- are most likely to lose sleep over work
- are most likely to feel they are workaholics

What Should We Do?

This book isn't about dieting. In fact, I believe we should avoid the word *dieting* altogeter. Fast food, cookies and chips aren't poison—unless we eat them in greater quantities than is healthy and are motivated to over eat based on marketing induced whims. Remember these keys:

- No one says you can't eat a little fat; just don't eat a lot. Eat something sweet; but not every day.
- We should also trust that Mother Nature got it right the first time, before we started stripping away the nutrients.

Then there's the question of cost. Snack and fast foods are cheap, while wholesome foods—the kinds found in health food stores—are expensive. Although it's true we pay more for these foods, I think it's worth it. Have you priced a colon resection lately?

The Common Thread

In previous chapters, I described all the vitamins, minerals and other food components we need for our health. Single-nutrient advice can be complicated and frustrating. People think, "I have to worry about calcium. I have to worry about folate. I have to worry about protein. I have to keep track of these forty different nutrients, and I'm confused." Don't be. My whole point was to show you what foods contain the nutrients and what current research shows us what they can do for us.

Some time in the future, possibly before you've started reading this book, another new thick RDA/DRI tome will be published. This one will be devoted to nutrition and disease. I don't know what the USDA and the National Academy of Sciences will say in the book; but I do know it will be confusing and much of the important data hard to find and understand.

Suffice it to say with this book, you will already have much of what you need. You want to increase your chances of warding off diseases such as cancer and heart disease? Eat whole grains and at least five servings of fruits and vegetables a day, even more if possible.

A Canadian study from the University of Toronto and St. Michael's Hospital and reported in the December 2002 issue of *Metabolism* found a combination diet of vegetables, nuts, soy proteins, and oats and barley can cut bad cholesterol by 29 percent, a reduction that matches the results of some drug treatments for high cholesterol.

Scientists have know for years that, individually, each of these food groups could lower cholesterol by 4–7 percent. However, this is the first study to look at this type of combination diet.

In the study, the researchers measured the cholesterol levels of thirteen people who went on a diet including vegetables such as broccoli, carrots, red peppers, tomato, onions, cauliflower, okra and eggplant. The diet also included oats, barley and psyllium; vegetable-based margarine; soy protein from products such as soy milk and soy sausages, cold cuts and burgers; and almonds.

In another study at about the same time, researchers found men who eat a diet that is rich in garlic, onions and scallions might also ward off prostate cancer. The Associated Press reports that new research from the National Cancer Institute points to men in China, who eat lots of garlic, scallions and onions as part of their regular diet, as having have the lowest rate of prostate cancer in the world.

For their study, the NCI researchers went to Shanghai, China, and interviewed 238 men who had prostate cancer and 471 men who did not, asking them how frequently they ate 122 food items. The results: Those who ate more than one-third of an ounce a day of garlic, onions or scallions—called the allium food group—cut in half their risk of prostate cancer. And the link is very strong, independent of body size, other foods eaten and total calories consumed.

Lead author Ann W. Hsing cautioned that the study results need to be replicated. Still, the results are stunning. Scallions offered the most protection: Those who ate just a tenth of an ounce daily reduced their prostate risk by about 70 percent. Garlic dropped the risk by 53 percent. In practical terms, Hsing advises men to eat one clove of garlic a day.

Same Old, Same Old . . .

Do you think eating the same old fruits vegetables and grains will get boring? Experiment with fruits you've never tried or thought you didn't like. There are literally hundreds of choices. For example, when was the last time you drank grape juice? A recent research study found that drinking Concord grape juice slowed the oxidation of LDL in the body, which, according to the study's author, Ishwarlal Jialal, M.D., Ph.D., Professor, Department of Pathology and Internal Medicine, University of California-Davis, could complement LDL reduction in the battle for a healthy heart.

"We know that high levels of LDL cholesterol in the body contribute to heart disease," said Dr. Jialal. "Taking steps to impede the oxidation of LDL is a complementary pathway to cardiovascular health." The study appeared in the December 2002 issue of the *American Journal of Clinical Nutrition*.

What about whole grains? Do you think you would get tired of brown rice, couscous or orzo any quicker than you can say Uncle Ben's? Consider quinoa (pronounced *keen-wa*), a grain originating in the Andes Mountains of South America. Quinoa was one of the three staple foods, along with corn and potatoes, of the Inca civilization.

Quinoa contains more protein than any other grain; an average of 16.2 percent, compared with 7.5 percent for rice, 9.9 percent for millet and 14 percent for wheat. Some varieties of quinoa are more than 20 percent protein. Quinoa's protein is a complete protein with an essential amino acid balance. Quinoa's protein is high in lysine, methionine and cystine. This makes it an excellent food to combine with, and boost the protein value of, other grains (which are low in lysine), or soy (which is low in methionine and cystine). Quinoa is only one example; there are dozens of other grains you probably never heard of but are available in health food and ethnic markets.

The Bottom Line

Regardless of government nutritional guidelines, and despite the influence of outside parties and marketing efforts of the food companies, the bottom line is there is only one person who should be influencing our eating habits—both good and bad. You know this person well; in fact he or she is in the room right now holding and reading this very book.

You are not average—don't let anyone tell you so. Your body—at your age, at your activity level, at your weight—has nutrient needs that probably are very different from the nutrient needs of the government's prescribed "average person." Remember that. The resources to help you find a better way to treat your body are out there. Find them and follow them closely. Hopefully, this book will be at the top of the stack.

References

Chapters 1 and 2

Atwater, W.O.; Farmers' Bulletin, U.S. Department of Agriculture, 1894.

Atwater, Hunt; How to Select Foods, USDA, 1917.

Hunt, Caroline; Food for Young Children, USDA, 1916.

Milton, Katherine, International Journal of Basic and Applied Nutritional Sciences, June 1999.

Milton, K., "Nutritional characteristics of wild Primate foods: Do the natural diets of our closest living relatives have lessons for us?" Nutrition 15(6) 1999.

Nestle, Marion; Food Politics, University of California Press, 2002.

Jacob Selhub, Ph.D., Paul F. Jacques, Sc.D., Andrew G. Bostom, M.D., Ralph B. D'Agostino, Ph.D., Peter W.F. Wilson, M.D., Albert J. Belanger, M.A., Daniel H. O'Leary, M.D., Philip A. Wolf, M.D., Ernst J. Schaefer, M.D., and Irwin H. Rosenberg, M.D. "Association between Plasma Homocysteine Concentrations and Extracranial Carotid-Artery Stenosis" The New England Journal of Medicine February 2, 1995; Volume 332:286-291.

Quatromoni, Dr. Paula A., "Dietary patterns predict the development of overweight in women: The Framingham Nutrition studies" Journal of the American Dietetic Association, September 2002

USDA and Academy of Science Documents

"Dietary Reference Intakes for Calcium, Phosphorus, Magnesium, Vitamin D, and Fluoride," Food and Nutrition Board, Institute of Medicine, 1999.

Dietary Reference Intakes: A Risk Assessment Model for Establishing Upper Intake Levels for Nutrients, Food and Nutrition Board, Institute of Medicine, National Academy of Science, National Academies Press, 1999.

Dietary Reference Intakes for Vitamin C, Vitamin E, Selenium, and Carotenoids, Food and Nutrition Board, Institute of Medicine, National Academy of Science, National Academies Press, 2000.

Dietary Reference Intakes for Thiamin, Riboflavin, Niacin, Vitamin B6, Folate, Vitamin B12, Pantothenic Acid, Biotin, and Choline, Food and Nutrition Board, Institute of Medicine, National Academy of Science, National Academies Press, 2000.

Dietary Reference Intakes: Applications in Dietary Assessment, Food and Nutrition Board, Institute of Medicine, National Academy of Science, National Academies Press, 2001.

Dietary Reference Intakes for Vitamin A, Vitamin K, Arsenic, Boron, Chromium, Copper, Iodine, Iron, Manganese, Molybdenum, Nickel, Silicon, Vanadium, and Zinc, Food and Nutrition Board, Institute of Medicine, National Academy of Science, National Academies Press, 2002.

Dietary Reference Intakes for Energy, Carbohydrate, Fiber, Fat, Fatty Acids, Cholesterol, Protein, and Amino Acids, Food and Nutrition Board, Institute of Medicine, National Academy of Science, National Academies Press, 2002.

Websites:

Council for Responsible Nutrition www.crnusa.org

Food and Nutrition Board (FNB) of the National Academy of Sciences (NAS) www.iom.edu/IOM/IOMHome.nsf/Pages/About+FNB

National Health and Nutrition Examination Survey www.cdc.gov/nchs/nhanes.htm

Physicians Committee for Responsible Medicine www.pcrm.org

US Department of Agriculture (USDA) www.usda.gov

Western Human Nutrition Research Center www.whnrc.usda.gov

Chapters 3 and 4

American Gastroenterological Association, "Obesity Guidelines," Gastroenterology, September 2002.

Bero LA, Galbraith A, Rennie D., "The publication of sponsored symposiums in medical journals," N Engl J Med, 1992;327:1135-1140.

Blackburn, George L. M.D., "The American Obesity Epidemic Is Getting Worse," FOOD TECHNOLOGY, JUNE 2002.

Blumenthal D, Campbell EG, Anderson MS, et al., "Withholding research results in academic life science," JAMA 1997;277:1224-1228.

Boyd EA, Bero LA., "Assessing faculty financial relationships with industry: a case study," JAMA 2000;284:2209-2214.

Brook, Yaron, Alex Epstein, "Equal Time: New rules hamstring businesses (Editorial)" Atlanta Journal and Constitution, October 2002.

"Caffeine, genes tied to bone loss in older women" Health eLine, Reuters Health, October 25, 2001.

Cohen R. "Conference call," New York Times, September 24, 2000: Magazine section:30-32.

Finke, Michael S.,Ph.D., Connie Diekman, M.Ed., R.D., L.D., F.A.D.A., American Dietetic Association; Family and Consumer Sciences Research Journal, December 2002.

Fit for Life, The Sugar Association, Inc., Washington, DC 2002.

Flegal, Katherine M.; Margaret D. Carroll; Cynthia L. Ogden; Clifford L. Johnson, "Prevalence and Trends in Obesity Among US Adults, 1999-2000,," JAMA 2002; October 9, 2002 288:1723-1727.

Fontanarosa, Phil B., MD, "Editorial: Obesity Research, A Call for Papers," JAMA 2002, October 9, 2002.

Green, Valerie, "Introducing the New Food Pyramid;Researchers Believe There is a Better Way to Eat," Tufts Daily, October 1, 2001.

Hu, Frank B. M.D., Meir J. Stampfer, M.D., JoAnn E. Manson, M.D., Eric Rimm, Sc.D., Graham A. Colditz, M.D., Bernard A. Rosner, Ph.D., Charles H. Hennekens, M.D., and Walter C. Willett, M.D., "Dietary Fat Intake and the Risk of Coronary Heart Disease in Women," New England Journal of Medicine, Nov 20, 1997, 337:1491-1499.

Lee, Elizabeth, "Eating more fruits, veggies gets push." Atlanta Journal and Constitution, September 23, 2002.

McCook, Alison, "Caffeine, even in small doses, may hurt arteries," Health eLine 2002-05-17Reuters Health on May 21, 2002 temporary stiffening of the blood vessel walls

McCook, Alison, "Caffeine boosts stress level all day long: study Health eLine 2002-07-30

Milloy, Steven, "New Nutrition Book Choking on Bad Science," FOXNews.com, February 22, 2002.

National Research Council, Report of the Committee on Diet and Health, Food and Nutrition Board, Commission on Life Sciences. Diet and health: implications for reducing chronic disease risk. Washington, DC: National Academy Press;1989.

Patterson BH, Block G, Rosenberger WF, Pee D, Kahle LL. Fruit and veg-etables in the American diet: data from the NHANES II Survey. American Journal of Public Health, 1990; 80(12):1443-9.

Russell, Robert M., Helen Rasmussen and Alice H. Lichtenstein, "Modified Food Guide Pyramid for People over Seventy Years of Age," Journal of Nutrition, March 1999;129:751-753.)

Schllosser, Eric, Fast Food Nation, Houghton Mifflin, 2001.

Shell, Ellen Ruppel, The Hungry Gene: The Science of Fat and the Future of Thin, Atlantic Monthly Press, 2002.

U.S. Department of Agriculture. The food guide pyramid. Washington, DC:

U.S. Department of Agriculture. Home and Garden Bulletin No. 252, 1992. 40.

U.S. Department of Agriculture. Human Nutrition Information Service: Nationwide Food Consumption Survey, Continuing Survey of Food Intakes by Individuals: Women 19-50 Years and Their Children 1-5 Years, 1 Day, 1985. Washington, DC: USDA. Report No. 85-1, 1986.

U.S. Department of Agriculture. Human Nutrition Information Service: Nationwide Food Consumption Survey, Continuing Survey of Food Intakes by Individuals: Women 19-50 Years and Their Children 1-5 Years, 1 Day, 1986. Washington, DC: U.S. Department of Agriculture. Report No. 86-1, 1987.

U.S. Department of Health and Human Services. The Surgeon General's report on nutrition and health. Washington, DC: U.S. Department of Health and Human Services, U.S. Public Health Service, Office of the Surgeon General. 1988; DHHS Publication No. (PHS) 88-50210.

Willett, Walter, Eat Drink and be Healthy, Harvard School of Public Health, 2002.

Websites:

American Council on Science and Health, Inc. (ACSH) www.acsh.org

American Obesity Association www.obesity.org/

Centers for Disease Control and Prevention www.cdc.gov

Center For Consumer Freedom (CCF) www.CCF.org

Center for Science in the Public Interest (CSPI) www.cspinet.org

Food Policy Institute at the Consumer Federation of America www.consumerfed.org

Harvard School of Public Health Nutrition Source www.hsph.harvard.edu/nutritionsource/

International Food Information Council Foundation (IFIC) www.ific.org/food

Steven Milloy www.JunkScience.com

National Food Processors Association www.nfpa-food.org

National Institutes of Health www.nih.gov

National Restaurant Association www.restaurant.org

The Nurses' Health Study (Harvard Medical School, Harvard School of Public Health, Brigham and Women's Hospital, Dana Farber Cancer Institute, Boston Children's Hospital and Beth Israel Hospital.) www.nurseshealthstudy.org

Public Citizen www.citizen.org

Chapter 5

Cauchon D., "FDA advisers tied to industry," USA Today. September 25, 2000:01A.

Cho MK, Shohara R, Schissel A, Rennie D., "Policies on faculty conflicts of interest at US universities," JAMA 2000;284:2203-2208.

Davis R. Health education on the six-o'clock news. Motivating television coverage of news in medicine. JAMA 1988;259(7):1036-8.

Davis C and Saltos E. Dietary recommendations and how they have changed over time. In: Elizabeth Frazao, America's eating habits: changes and consequences. Washington, DC: U.S. Department of Agriculture, Food and Rural Economics Division. Agriculture Information Bulletin No. 750, 1999. p. 33-50.

Guidelines for communicating emerging science on nutrition, food safety and health. J Natl Cancer Inst 1998;90(3):194-9.

Kassirer J.P., "Financial indigestion," JAMA, 2000;284:2156-2157.

Kaufman L. Prime-time nutrition. J Communication 1990;30(3):37-45.

Korn D., "Conflicts of interest in biomedical research," JAMA 2000; 284:2234-2237.

Levy AL, Stokes R. Effects of a health promotion advertising campaign on sales of ready-to-eat cereals. Public Health Rep 1987;102:398-403.

Nelkin D. An uneasy relationship: the tensions between medicine and the media. Lancet 1996;347(9015):1600-3.

Peterson M., "What's black and white and sells medicine?" New York Times. August 27, 2000; sect 3:1.

Rochon P., "Evaluating the quality of articles published in journal supplements compared with the quality of those published in the parent journal," JAMA, 1994;272:108-113.

Russo JE, Staelin R, Nolan CA, Russell GJ, Metcalf BL. Nutrition information in the supermarket. J Consumer Res 1986;13(1):48-70.

Website:

National consumer survey confirms: Americans flip-flop on food choices when nutrition studies conflict. December 9, 1999. www.margarine.org/pr13.html

Chapters 6 and 7

Baranowski T, Davis M, Resnicow K, Baranowski J, Doyle C, Smith M, Lin LS, Smith M, Wang DT. Gimme 5 fruit, juice, and vegetables for fun and health: outcome evaluation. Health Educ Behav 2000;27(1):96-111.

Costain, Lyndel, Super Nutrients Handbook, Dk Pub Merchandise, 2001

Dietary Reference Intakes for Energy, Carbohydrate, Fiber, Fat, Fatty Acids, Cholesterol, Protein, and Amino Acids, Food and Nutrition Board, Institute of Medicine, National Academy of Science, National Academies Press, 2002.

Feskanich D, Willett WC, Stampfer MJ, Colditz GA. Protein consumption and bone fractures in women. Am J Epidemiol 1996; 143:472-9.

Hightower, Jane, MD, Environmental Health Perspectives, November 2002.

Hu FB, Stampfer MJ, Manson JE, et al. Dietary protein and risk of ischemic heart disease in women. Am J Clin Nutr 1999; 70:221-7.

Ingram, Colin, The Drinking Water Book: A Complete Guide to Safe Drinking Water, Ten Speed Press, 1991.

Jensen, Michael, MD, NORTH AMER ASSOC STUDY OBESITY, MAYO
MEDICAL CENTER, MAYO CLIN200 FIRST ST, SWROCHESTER,
MN, 55905

Krebs-Smith SM, Kantor LS. Choose a variety of fruits and vegetables daily:
understanding the complexities. Journal of Nutrition, 2000;131.

Lewis, Scott Alan, The Sierra Club Guide to Safe Drinking Water, Sierra
Club Books, 1996.

Li R, Serdula M, Bland S, Mokdad A, Bowman B, Nelson D. Trends in fruit
and vegetable consumption among adults in 16 U.S. states: Behavioral
Risk Factor Surveillance System, 1990-1996, Am J Public Health
2000;90(5):777-81.

Perry CL, Bishop DB, Taylor G, Murray DM, Mays RW, Dudovitz BS,
Smyth M, Story M. Changing fruit and vegetable consumption among
children: the 5 A Day Power Plus Program in St. Paul, Minnesota. Am J
Public Health. 1998;88(4):603-9.

Shipman JT. An introduction to Physical Science. Boston , MA: Houghton
Mifflin Co., 2002.

Spreen, Alan M., MD, CNC, Nutritionally Incorrect, Woodland Publishing,
2002.

USDA Nutrient Database for Standard Reference, Release 14. US
Department of Agriculture. accessed on 18 July 2002.

Valtin, Heinz, MD, American Journal of Physiology Aug 8, 2002.

Websites:
Ball State University News Center, www.bsu.edu/news
Dartmouth-Hitchcock Medical Center, www.dartmouth.edu/dms/news

Chapter 8

Phyllis A., C.N.C. Balch, James F., M.D. Balch, Prescription for Nutritional
Healing: A Practical A-Z Reference to Drug-Free Remedies Using
Vitamins, Minerals, Herbs, and Food Supplements, Avery Penguin
Putnam. 2000.

Hass, Elton M., Staying Healthy With Nutrition: The Complete Guide to
Diet and Nutritional Medicine, Celestial Arts, 1992.

The Healing Power of Vitamins, Minerals, and Herbs:
The A-Z Guide to Enhancing Your Health and Treating Illness with
Nutritional Supplements, Reader's Digest Association, 1999.

Mindell, Earl, Earl Mindell's Vitamin Bible for the 21st Century, Warner
Books, 1999.

National Cancer Institute. Diet, nutrition, and cancer prevention: a guide
to food choices. Bethesda, MD: National Institutes of Health, National
Cancer Institute. 1984; NIH Publication No. 85-2711.

Websites:
Crohn's & Colitis Foundation of America, Inc.: www.ccfa.org/

New York Times www.nytimes.com
Nutrient Database for Standard Reference, Release 15 (SR15)
    http://www.nal.usda.gov/fnic/foodcomp/Data/SR15/sr15.html

Chapter 9, 10 and 11

Alpha-Tocopherol, Beta Carotene Cancer Prevention Study Group. The effect of vitamin E and beta carotene on the incidence of lung cancer and other cancers in male smokers. New England Journal of Medicine 330:1029-1035, 1994.

American Journal of Epidemiology 2002;156:274-285.

American Journal of Respiratory and Critical Care Medicine, May 2002

Anderson JW, Johnstone BM, Cook-Newell ME. Meta-analysis of the effects of soy protein intake on serum lipids, N Engl J Med 1995; 333:276-82.

Balch, James F., M.D, The Super Anti-Oxidants: Why They Will Change the Face of Healthcare in the 21st Century, M Evans & Co, 1999.

Beling, Stephanie, Powerfoods: Good Food, Good Health With Phytochemicals, Nature's Own Energy Boosters, HarperCollins, 1998.

Bland, Jeffrey, Earl Mindell, Bioflavoniods, Keats Publishing, 1984.

Block, Gladys, MD, American Journal of Epidemiology, June 2002, p224

Block G., Dietary guidelines and the results of food consumption surveys. Am J Clin Nutr. 1991;53(suppl): 356S-357S.

Byers T, Perry G. Dietary carotenes, vitamin C, and vitamin E as protective antioxidants in human cancers. Ann Rev Nutr. 1992;12: 139-159.

Jack Challam, Smith, Melissa Diane, User's Guide to Vitamin E: Don't Be a Dummy: Become an Expert on What Vitamin E Can Do for Your Health, Basic Health Publications, Inc., 2002.

de Haan JB and others. Reactive oxygen species and their contribution to pathology in Down syndrome. Advances in Pharmacology 38:379-402, 1997.

Dicyan, Erwin, Passwater, Richard, "Beginner's Introduction to Trace Minerals, Keats Publishing, 1984.

Dwyer, James H. Ph.D., Circulation, June 19, 2001.

Elkins, Rita, Soy Smart Health: Discover the 'Super Food' That Fights Breast Cancer, Heart Disease, Osteoporosis, Menopausal Discomforts, and Estrogen Dominance, Woodland Publishing, 2000.

Goodman, Sandra, Vitamin C: The Master Nutrient, Keats Publishing, 1992.

Erdman JW, Jr. "AHA Science Advisory: Soy protein and cardiovascular disease: A statement for healthcare professionals from the Nutrition Committee of the AHA," Circulation 2000; 102:2555-9.

Greenberg ER, Baron JA, Tosteson TD, Freeman DH, Beck GJ, Bond JH, Colacchio TA, Coller JA, Frankl HD, Haile RW. A clinical trial of antioxidant vitamins to prevent colo-rectal adenoma. New Engl J Med. 1994;331:141-147.

Gutterodge, John M., Bary Halliwell, Antioxidants in Nutrition, Health, and Disease, Oxford University Press, 1995.

"Health claims: Soy protein and risk of coronary heart disease," Code of
   Federal Regulations, 21CFR101.82 (2001).
Hatherill, J. Robert, Eat to Beat Cancer, Renaissance Books, 1999.
Hay, Jennifer, Vitamin C: Everything You Need to Know, Peoples Medical
   Society, 1998.
Hennekens CH and others. Antioxidant vitamins: Benefits not yet proved.
   New England Journal of Medicine 330:1080-1081, 1994.
Hoffer, Abram, M.D., Linus Pauling, Vitamin C & Cancer: Discovery,
   Recovery, Controversy, Quarry Pressm 2001.
Kurl, Sudhir, MD, Stroke: Journal of the American Heart Association, June
   2002.
LeBars, et al. "A Placebo-Controlled, Double-Blind, Randomized Trial of an
   Extract of Ginkgo Biloba for Dementia." JAMA. 1997; 278(16): 1327-1332.
Meskin, Mark S., (Editor), Phytochemicals in Nutrition and Health,
   Technomic Pub Co., 2002.
Messina M, Gardner C, Barnes S., "Gaining insight into the health effects
   of soy but a long way still to go: commentary on the fourth International
   Symposium on the Role of Soy in Preventing and Treating Chronic
   Disease," Journal of Nutrition 2002; 132:547S-551S.
Moyad, Mark A., MPH, The ABC's of Nutrition & Supplements for
   Prostate Cancer, Sleeping Bear Press, 2000.
Omenn GS and others. Effects of a combination of beta carotene and vita-
   min A on lung cancer and cardiovascular disease. New England Journal
   of Medicine 334:1150-1155, 1996.
Oyama, et al. "Ginkgo biloba extract protects brain neurons against oxida-
   tive stress induced by hydrogen peroxide." Brain Research. 1996;
   712:349-352.
Pierpaoli, Walter, MD, Regelson, William MD, The Melatonin Miracle, G K
   Hall & Co, 1996.
Prinzenberg, Ernst D., Ginseng: Stay Young and Vital, Sterling
   Publications, 1999.
Reynolds RD. Vitamin supplements: current controversies. J Am Coll Nutr.
   1994;13(2): 118-126.
Ruihai, Liu, Journal of Agriculture and Food Chemistry, Aug. 14, 2002.
Rimm EB and others. Vitamin consumption and the risk of coronary dis-
   ease in men. New England Journal of Medicine 328:1450-1456, 1993.
Shultz, Clifford W., MD, COQ10, Archives of Internal Medicine, October
   2002.
Stampfer MJ and others. Vitamin consumption and the risk of coronary dis-
   ease in women. New England Journal of Medicine 328:1444-1449, 1993.
Tribble DL and others. Antioxidant consumption and risk of coronary
   heart disease: Emphasis on vitamin C, vitamin E, and beta-carotene.
   American Heart Association Science Advisory. Circulation 99:591-595,
   1999.
Weisburger JH. Nutritional approach to cancer prevention with emphasis
   on vitamins, antioxidants, and carotenoids. Am J Clin Nutr.
   1991;53(suppl): 226S-237S

White LR, Petrovitch H, Ross GW, et al, "Brain aging and midlife tofu consumption," J Am Coll Nutr 2000; 19:242-55.

Wurtman, Richard, "Carbohydrates and Depression,." Scientific American, January 1989.

Ziegler, RG. Vegetables, fruits, and carotenoids and the risk of cancer. Am J Clin Nutr 1991;53(1 suppl):251S-259S.

Websites:

American Cancer Society www.cancer.org
American Journal of Clinical Nutrition www.ajcn.org
National Sleep Foundation (NSF) www.sleepfoundation.org
National Cancer Insitute www.nci.nih.gov/
QuackWatch www.quackwatch.com
Univ. of California Berkeley's Wellness Letter www.berkeleywellness.com

Chapter 12 and 13

The Merck Manual, Sec. 1, Ch. 3, Vitamin Deficiency, Dependency, And Toxicity, 1995-2002 Merck & Co., Inc.,

Reavley, Nicola, The New Encyclopedia of Vitamins, Minerals, Supplements, & Herbs, M Evans & Co., 1999.

Ursell, Amanda, Vitamins & Minerals Handbook, Dk Pub Merchandise, 2001.

Varosy, Paul D., MD, 42nd annual conference on Cardiovascular Disease and Epidemiology Prevention in Honolulu, Hawaii.

Wasmuth HE, Kolb H. "Cow's milk and immune-mediated diabetes," Proc Nutr Soc 2000; 59:573-9

Weil, Andrew, Eating Well for Optimum Health: The Essential Guide to Food, Diet, and Nutrition, Alfred A. Knopf, 2000.

Willett WC. "Vitamin A and lung cancer," Nutrition Review 1990; 48(5):201-11.

Websites:

American Academy of Pediatrics www.aap.org
Creighton University in Omaha (Robert Heaney, MD) www.medicine.creighton.edu/medschool/medicine/
Institute of Shortening and Edible Oils www.iseo.org
Lloyd, Thomas, PhD American Journal of Public Health, June 1997.
Rockefeller University in New York www.rockefeller.edu
USDA Human Nutrition Research Center on Aging at Tufts University in Boston www.library.tufts.edu/hnrc/hnrc.html
Weill Medical College of Cornell University www.med.cornell.edu

Chapter 14

American Cancer Society 1996 Advisory Committee on Diet, Nutrition, and Cancer prevention, Guidelines on diet, nutrition, and cancer prevention: reducing the risk of cancer with healthy food choices and physical activity, The American Cancer Society 1996 Advisory Committee on Diet, Nutrition, and Cancer Prevention, CA Cancer J Clin 1996;46(6):325-41.

Gallo A. Food advertising in the United States. In: Elizabeth Frazao, America's eating habits: changes and consequences, Washington, DC: U.S. Department of Agriculture. Agricultural Information Bulletin No. 750. 1999. p. 173-80.

Glanz K, Basil M, Maibach E, Goldberg J, Snyder D. Why Americans eat what they do: taste, nutrition, cost, convenience, and weight control concerns are influences on food consumption. J Am Diet Assoc 1998; 98(10):1118-26.

Horne PJ, Lowe CF, Fleming PF, Dowey AJ. An effective procedure for changing food preferences in 5-7-year-old children. Proc Nutr Soc 1995;54(2):441-52.

Horne PJ, Lowe CF, Bowdery M, Egerton C., "The way to healthy eating for children," Br Food J 1998;100(3): 133-40.

Jialal, Ishwarlal, MD, American Journal of Clinical Nutrition, December 2002.

Reynolds KD, Franklin FA, Brinkley D, Raczynski JM, Harrington KF, Kirk KA, Person S., "Increasing the fruit and vegetable consumption of fourth graders: results from the High 5 project," Prev Med, 2000;30(4): 309-19.

U.S. Department of Agriculture, Agricultural Research Service, Dietary Guidelines Advisory Committee, Report of the Dietary Guidelines Advisory Committee on the dietary guidelines for Americans, 1995.

U.S. Department of Agriculture, Agricultural Research Service, Dietary Guidelines Advisory Committee: Report of the Dietary Guidelines Advisory Committee on the dietary guidelines for Americans, 2000 To the Secretary of Agriculture and the Secretary of Health and Human Services. U.S. Department of Agriculture, Committee by the Agricultural Research Service, Dietary Guidelines Advisory Committee; 2000. 79 p.

World Cancer Research Fund and the American Institute for Cancer Research, Food, Nutrition and the Prevention of Cancer: a Global Perspective, Washington, DC: American Institute for Cancer Research, 1997.

Websites:
American Heart Association www.amhrt.org
Oxford Health Plans www.oxhp.com

Index

About the Author

Mike Fillon has written about health and medical topics for more than 15 years. For *Popular Mechanics,* he has written over 400 articles on a broad variety of medical, technological, and scientific subjects. Recently he wrote six cover stories—including two articles for two of the top-selling issues in the magazine's 100-year history. Mr. Fillon has written more than 150 consumer-oriented news and feature stories for WebMD, CBS HealthWatch, MSNBC, and the *Reader's Digest* Web sites. He has written both short and feature-length pieces for more than two dozen other publications, including *Health Week, NCN News*—a Novartis Pharmaceutical newsletter—*Information Week* and *Science Digest.* He has also written for the American Cancer Society, Emory University and the Center for Disease Control and Prevention (CDC). Additionally, he has been interviewed on numerous radio shows and has appeared on the *Weekend Today Show* and *American Morning with Paula Zahn.*

Mr. Fillon has recently published two very successful health booklets: *Conquering Caffeine Dependence* and *Conquering Food Triggers.* He also had two books published in 1999: *Natural Prostate Healers,* by Prentice Hall, and *Young Superstars of Tennis,* for Avisson Press. He also contributed a number of chapters for the *Reader's Digest* title *Looking After Your Body.* He wrote sections on shingles, problems of the gall bladder, thyroid, prostate, back problems, and a wide range of gastrointestinal illnesses.

Mr. Fillon has a Master of Science degree of the State University of New York Maritime College. He is a member of the American Medical Writer's Association and the National Association of Science Writers.

Mr. Fillon lives in Atlanta with his wife, Sue, their children Sarah, Emilie and Evan, and a golden retriever named Sandy Koufax.